KIM BOYCE
Beauty
TO LAST A LIFETIME

with Ken Abraham

CHARIOT
FAMILY PUBLISHING

Chariot Family Publishing is a division of David C. Cook Publishing Co.
David C. Cook Publishing Co., Elgin, Illinois 60120
David C. Cook Publishing Co., Weston, Ontario
Nova Distribution Ltd., Newton Abbot, England

BEAUTY TO LAST A LIFETIME: A STEP BY STEP GUIDE TO INNER AND OUTER BEAUTY FOR
TEENAGE GIRLS
© 1992 by Kim Boyce with Ken Abraham for text and Sarah Johnson for illustrations

Unless otherwise noted, Scripture quotations are from New American Standard Bible, © the
Lockman Foundation 1960, 1962, 1963, 1968, 1971, 1972, 1973, 1975, 1977.

Scripture quotations marked (NIV) are from the Holy Bible, New International Version, © 1973,
1978, 1984, International Bible Society; used by permission of Zondervan Bible Publishers.

Verses marked (TLB) are taken from The Living Bible, © 1971, Tyndale House Publishers,
Wheaton, IL 60189. Used by permission.

Scripture quotations marked (KJV) are from the King James Version.

Unless otherwise noted, all quotations in the margins are reprinted from *Quotable Quotations*,
compiled by Lloyd Cory, published by Victor Books, 1985, SP Publications, Inc. Wheaton IL 60187.

Designed by Helen Lannis
Photography by Marshall Arts
Makeup by Lori Cohn. Represented by David and Lee, Chicago.
Models: Christy McCarthy and Jennifer Mosses.
First Printing, 1992
Printed in the United States of America
96 95 94 93 92   5 4 3 2 1

Library of Congress Cataloging-in-Publication Data

Boyce, Kim.
Beauty to last a lifetime : a step by step guide to inner and outer beauty for teenage girls / by
Kim Boyce and Ken Abraham.
          p.   cm.
Summary: offers advice on such topics as skin and hair care, tanning, weight control, exercise,
and makeup, with a Christian perspective.
ISBN 0-7814-0988-8
1. Teenage girls—Health and hygiene. 2. Beauty, Personal.
[1. Beauty, Personal. 2. Grooming. 3. Health. 4. Christian life.]
I. Abraham, Ken. II. Title.
RA777.25.B68   1992
646.7'042—dc20   92-12611
                                                                      CIP
                                                                      AC

CONTENTS

Read Me First!

INNER BEAUTY? YOU MAY BE WONDERING. What in the world is that? Where does it come from? How can I develop my own? I'm having enough problems trying to get my external "look" together, and you want me to develop inner beauty as well? Yes! I do! But don't worry; it won't be a hassle. It will be fun.

External beauty is such an ambiguous quality; trying to figure it out is like grasping at fog. Styles come and go; trends concerning

There are two kinds of beauty. There is a beauty which God gives at birth, and which withers as a flower. And there is a beauty which God grants when by His grace men are born again. That kind of beauty never vanishes but blooms eternally.

ABRAHAM KUYPER

our personal appearance are in a constant state of transition. It's tough to even maintain a wardrobe that is semi up-to-date. By the time you save enough money to buy that special new outfit, the fashions have changed!

Perhaps that is why the Lord cautions us against basing our beauty on transient, external adornments. Instead, we are encouraged to pursue true beauty, "the hidden person of the heart, with the imperishable quality of a gentle and quiet spirit" (I Peter 3:4). That's what I am referring to in this book when I talk about qualities of "inner beauty."

The greatest part about inner beauty is that you don't have to develop it by yourself. In fact, you can't. You don't get up in the morning, brush your teeth, wash your face, put on your makeup, and then dab on a bit of inner beauty. It just doesn't work that way.

True inner beauty is the natural result of a relationship with Jesus Christ. It comes from knowing Him, trusting Him with your life, and allowing Him to live in and through you. In a real way, inner beauty is the result of the characteristics of Jesus shining out through your life.

But what is Jesus like? What are His personality traits that He wants to develop in you? The apostle Paul gave us one of the best descriptions of the character of Jesus when he listed "the fruit of the Spirit."

Check this out: "The fruit of the Spirit is love, joy, peace, patience, kindness, goodness, faithfulness, gentleness, self-control . . . " (Galatians 5:22, 23). Wow! Have you ever read a better description of the character of Jesus? Now, if Jesus' character is going to show up in your life as qualities of inner beauty, guess what traits are going to be evidenced. Yep! Love. Joy. Peace. And all the rest!

In this book, we'll spend a lot of time discussing how you can improve your external appearance, and how you can feel better about yourself. Most young women I meet nowadays are concerned about that. But the most important point I want you to understand is that true beauty, real and lasting beauty, the kind that lasts a lifetime, only comes from your inner relationship with Jesus.

That's why throughout these pages I'll be asking you some thought-provoking questions in the margins. I don't want to embarrass you or put you on the spot. I just want you to think about some of the things that I am convinced really matter in life. I'm hoping that these questions will help you understand the balance between external attractiveness and the eternal qualities of inner beauty. I'll also be giving you some Scripture verses that will, hopefully, help put things in perspective for you.

For example, one of my favorite verses in the Bible pertaining to beauty is a formula for successful femininity. It is not a list of dos and don'ts, but an attitude of the heart. "Charm is deceitful and beauty is vain, but a woman who fears the Lord, she shall be praised" (Proverbs 31:30).

A woman who fears the Lord (who has a reverential awe of God, sort of a "God Is Awesome" attitude), will have a radiant beauty about her even in the absence of artificial adornments such as makeup, jewelry, or designer clothing. This woman has respect for the person of God, the Word of God, and the things of God. As such, she has a healthy self-respect. She takes care of and develops the body and mind God has given her, knowing all the while that she doesn't need to be built like a fashion model or look like a movie star to be truly beautiful. The qualities of inner beauty won't fade away with time. They will last a lifetime . . . and beyond!

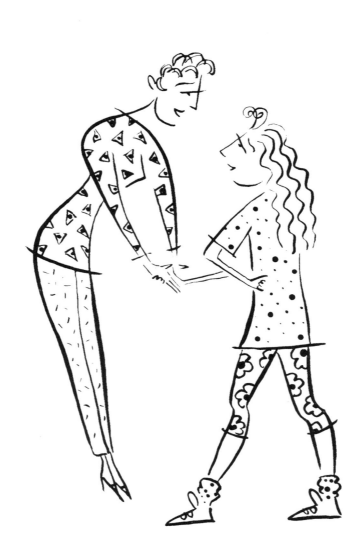

Getting Acquainted

BEING A YOUNG WOMAN TODAY IS MORE difficult and confusing than it has ever been before. It is also more challenging and exciting. You have options and opportunities that your mom and grandmother never even dreamed about! Along with those new possibilities comes the need for increased awareness, responsibility, and accountability. More than ever, you need to know who you are, and you need to genuinely like that person.

When I first considered writing this book, I must confess I had one major reservation. I was confident that I could—with a little help from some experts, and by drawing upon my own experiences from traveling and meeting thousands of teenage young women every year—answer most of the usual questions about beauty in a semi-intelligent and hopefully helpful manner. Still, I wondered whether I could write something that would have a deeper meaning, and not just give you some ideas about how to put on your makeup.

As I began the process of organizing my thoughts, it occurred to me that I really did have something important to say, not just about the nitty-gritty matters of dress and makeup, diet and exercise, but also about that wonderful, mysterious, often elusive quality of inner beauty. This book is my way of sharing with you some of what I've learned.

We are shaped and fashioned by what we love.
GOETHE

MY PERSONAL BEAUTY QUEST

I asked Jesus Christ to come into my life when I was only seven years old. I'll never forget it. I was attending a youth camp in central Florida. It wasn't a fancy camp with fabulous facilities and tons of things for us to do. It was plain and simple. The services were held in an old-fashioned, open-air tabernacle with dirt floors, and when the preacher instructed all those kids who wanted to ask Jesus to come into their hearts to come forward, I responded.

I was a little nervous and slightly scared—I didn't quite know what to expect when Jesus came into my heart—but I knew the preacher said that Jesus loved me just the way I was, and He wanted to be my best friend. So when the invitation was given, I stepped out of the aisle where I had been standing and walked toward the front to join the crowd of kids in the Florida heat and dirt.

I didn't experience any earthquakes or thunderclaps, but Jesus really did come into my heart. I soon began to study the Bible and learn how Jesus wants me to live, and later I began to learn what it means to be a woman of God.

One passage of Scripture, Proverbs 31, really fascinated me. It is the description of "an excellent wife." To me, she was the original biblical bionic bombshell! In just a few verses, the writer listed more than twenty-four qualities of this woman. Here are some of the highlights. The woman in Proverbs 31 is one who . . .

> *can be trusted (vs. 11).*
> *is a hard worker (vs. 13).*
> *is an adventurous shopper (vs. 14).*
> *is an early riser (vs. 15).*
> *is a wise investor (vs. 16).*
> *is a strong (healthy) woman (vs. 17).*
> *is a self-confident woman (vs. 18).*
> *is a night owl, too (vs. 18).*
> *is a fashion designer (vs. 19).*
> *has a heart of compassion (vs. 20).*
> *is married to a well-respected man (vs. 23).*
> *is an entrepreneur (vs. 24)*
> *has a positive attitude (vs. 25).*
> *speaks wisdom (vs. 26).*
> *has a family who appreciates her (vss. 28, 29).*

When I read that description, I thought out loud, "Wow! That's the kind of woman I want to be!" Ever since then, to me, that's what it has really meant to be "a beautiful woman."

When I was thirteen years old, I had a fascination with a different kind of beauty—outer beauty. I actually

Think of the silliest advertisement you've ever seen in a fashion magazine. What were the advertisers really trying to sell you?

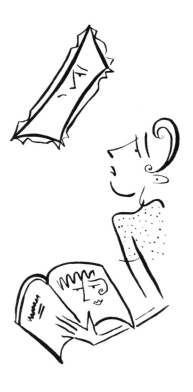

used to enjoy going to the orthodontist, because while sitting in the waiting room, I got to scour the various glamour magazines, most of which my parents didn't receive at home. As I pored over the latest issue of *Seventeen, Glamour,* or whatever else was available, I studied the articles as well as the pictures. I wanted to learn all I could about how to care for my body.

The beautiful women pictured on the pages were an enigma to me. I wondered, *How do those girls put their makeup on?* or, *What are they doing to themselves that causes them to look so good?* Little did I realize then, that those "pictures of perfection" gracing the magazine pages were impossible for me to duplicate in real life. The models in the magazines, the stars in television shows or in movies, or even your favorite music artists, rarely look as good in person as they do on film. The reason is obvious: they were made up for the camera and photographed with the best lighting equipment and camera angles available. Beyond that, the photos you finally see in the magazines are often retouched to make them look even better. You and I don't have that luxury in our everyday lives.

That's why it is such a waste of time, effort, and money to attempt to look like those celluloid images. You can't do it. When you try, you end up feeling worse about yourself because you can't achieve your goal. It's a no-win situation.

Unfortunately, nobody told me that when I was a teen. So there I was . . . sitting in front of Mom's makeup mirror with a glamour magazine in one hand and a tube of lipstick in the other, trying desperately to match my image in the mirror to the picture on the page. Some of my results were pretty outlandish, as you might guess.

Nevertheless, I had a lot of fun, and I did learn quite a bit about how to work with hair and makeup. I became so proficient at applying makeup and styling hair that by my mid-teens, I had earned a reputation at school for being the person with the answers when it came to beauty questions. Anytime my friends and I had a pajama party or stayed over at one another's homes, I loved to do everyone's hair and show them how to put on their makeup.

My best friend in high school was Jenny Campbell. When Jenny and I first met, she had an attractive appearance, clean and well-groomed. Jenny didn't wear any makeup and did little more with her hair than wash it, dry it, and comb it out. As we began hanging around together, Jenny became intrigued with how I did my makeup and hair. "Kim, how do you do that?" she'd ask in wide-eyed amazement. That was all the incentive I needed, and before long we were working on Jenny's new look. Within a year, Jenny was as good as or better than I was at doing makeup and hair.

What impresses you most when you meet a person for the first time? Personal appearance? Personality? Clothes?
Be specific.

BACKSTAGE AT THE MISS AMERICA PAGEANT

Just a few years later, I found myself thinking, *I don't believe I am doing this!* I was standing backstage at the Miss America Pageant at Convention Hall in Atlantic City. In a few moments, I was going to walk onto that stage and sing one of my favorite songs, "Somewhere Over the Rainbow," in front of an audience of nearly thirty thousand people. More than thirty million viewers were watching on television.

As I listened to the voice of Gary Collins, the popular television personality who was the master of ceremonies for the telecast, I took several deep breaths to calm last-minute jitters. It had been a nerve-racking week of competition, and I was as surprised as anyone when I was chosen as one of the top ten finalists. Now, the judges' scrutiny intensified as the Top Ten performed one last time prior to the selection of the new Miss America.

We had come to the talent competition, the area in which I felt most confident. But as I stood in the backstage shadows waiting for the contestant preceding me to complete her presentation, an awful thought struck me: *I wonder if the orchestra members will remember how to play my song!* I had not sung with the pageant orchestra since Wednesday evening during my preliminary talent presentation.

I didn't need to worry. The orchestra members were all tremendous musicians, and they had my song arrangements written out in front of them. *Still*, I kept wondering, *it has been four days since I have sung with them.* Practicing with my tape player and singing with a live orchestra are not exactly the same thing!

But time for fretting was gone. Gary Collins was introducing me: "Whatever the show, 'The Wizard of Oz' or 'The Muppet Movie,' it's always nice to have a rainbow song. And if one rainbow song makes a great ballad, a medley should be twice as nice. Here, putting 'Over the Rainbow' with 'The Rainbow Connection' is Kimberly Boyce, Miss Florida!"

The crowd applauded and I walked from my backstage mark to the center of the stage as the orchestra played a brief introduction. As soon as I began singing, I felt right at home. My nervousness fled away after the first line of the song; I relaxed and just enjoyed singing. It was fun! I had been singing in front of crowds for most of my life, and the Miss America Pageant audience was an enthusiastic one. They made it easy for me.

The Lord was preparing me to sing for Him long before I ever did my first solo concert. What special gift has He given to you? What might He be preparing you to do in the days ahead?

When I finished with the obligatory, Broadway-style ending, the audience applauded wildly. I raised my hands toward the sky as a gesture of thanks to the orchestra and whispered a short prayer of thanks to the Lord as I made my exit. There was nothing more to do now but wait until the talent competition was completed.

It seemed to take forever for the last few contestants to finish their talent presentations. I fidgeted nervously backstage all the while. Finally, the competition was over, the last commercial break had been taken, and the ten finalists were called on stage one more time.

Gary Collins began reading from his cue cards. I stood calmly with the nine other finalists as he announced the fourth runner-up, the third runner-up, and I was still standing there! Suddenly, the thought streaked through my mind, *I might have won this thing!* Not that I was confident of winning, but I had my preconceived ideas about who was going to win, and one by one those girls were being called out of line for lesser awards.

The second runner-up was number nine in the line of ten girls. I was number eight. Miss New York, number ten, was the only girl on my right.

Then Gary Collins announced the first runner-up— Suzette Charles, Miss New Jersey! Again the thought raced through my mind: *I seriously might have won this thing!*

Gary Collins's voice brought me back to reality.

"This is it!" he said into the cameras. "Our theme tonight has been 'Go for It,' and you'll agree these young women have given it everything. Now Miss America 1984 is about to be named. May I have the judges' decision, please?"

Our host walked across the stage to the front row

For God hath not given us the spirit of fear; but of power, and of love, and of a sound mind.

II TIMOTHY 1:7 (KJV)

If you compare yourself with others, you may become bitter or vain, for always there will be greater and lesser persons than yourself.

MAX EHRMANN

where the judges were seated. A distinguished looking, tuxedo-clad older gentleman stood up. He handed Gary Collins the envelope which contained the answer to the question everyone in the room was asking.

Collins walked briskly back to the microphone, pulling the card out of the envelope as he walked.

The last of the finalists stood on each side of Gary Collins. All five girls in my line gripped each other's hands tightly as we faced the audience. Our state banners had been removed. One of us would be walking off the stage wearing a new title—Miss America.

Gary Collins's strong voice sliced through the silence that had crept over the crowd. "And our new Miss America is . . . Vanessa Williams, Miss New York!"

His words echoed across the cavernous Convention Hall. A shriek pierced the air; then the entire auditorium erupted into applause, some sincerely expressed and some politely offered as part of protocol.

I turned to my right, and Vanessa and I spontaneously threw our arms around each other and hugged. Then the new Miss America turned on her heels and walked to the center of the stage, while I stood there applauding. Traces of tears moistened the corner of Vanessa's eyes, and she blinked them back as she accepted a beautiful bouquet of long-stemmed roses.

I stood in place, mechanically smiling and applauding the winner as all Miss America contestants are taught to do. About the time Vanessa was halfway down the runway, gliding gracefully to the tune of "There She Is . . . Miss America," it hit me. I lost . . . I lost this thing! I did not win.

Losing was a new sensation. I had never lost in a pageant before this. In every pageant I had ever entered (all four of them!), I had either been the first runner-up or the winner. But not here. I had lost. It was not a fun feeling, nor was it one I wanted to get used to, but it was one I had to accept. I stood empty-handed on the stage in front of millions of people.

Nevertheless, I learned a lot by entering the Miss Florida and Miss America Pageants. I learned what it means to be a winner, to have everybody pat you on the back and tell you how successful you are. And I experienced the pain of losing, the accompanying sense of insecurity and isolation, and the wondering whether anyone, other than your immediate loved ones, knows or cares if you exist.

I learned and now know that beauty is much more than "skin deep." It is being the best person I can be for God's glory, which does include looking and feeling my best. The key word there is <u>my</u>. I now know that I am only in competition with myself. What looks and feels right for me may not work for you. That's okay. You've got to go with what helps you to feel the best about you.

Being beautiful is not fitting into or filling out a certain dress size, nor is it having "perfect" teeth, hair, a "perfect" complexion, or skin tone. Real beauty starts on the inside and works its way out. It starts with a sense of peace and joy that comes from knowing that Jesus Christ loves and accepts me just the way I am. That puts a bounce in my step and a smile on my face, even when my hair is a mess or my face breaks out right before an important photo session.

If you are unhappy on the inside, no matter what you do to cover, color, or contour your external appearance, sooner or later, like the inevitable pimple that pops out at the worst times, the truth will surface.

On the other hand, if you know that God loves and accepts you exactly as you are, you can love and accept

Jesus says, "I love you just the way you are. And I love you too much to let you stay the way you are."

CHRIS LYONS

yourself and enjoy being the person He created you to be. When you know that your past mistakes, failures, and sins are forgiven, you can confidently step into the future unencumbered by a lot of the excess baggage that comes with a poor self-image, a negative attitude, or stubborn disobedience to God's plan for your life.

We all need an inner beauty—a beauty that begins on the inside and can't help but work its way out, a beauty that comes from knowing and accepting God's unconditional love. When you have that, whether the world ever acknowledges it or not, you are truly a beautiful person.

A BIT ABOUT ME

Before we go any further and get into outer beauty, let me fill you in a little about who I am and what credentials I have that might make me feel competent to comment upon your cut, comb, coiffure, and cuticle.

As a contemporary Christian music artist, I travel thousands of miles doing concerts in the United States as well as in several other countries. I meet a lot of kids every year. I love to talk personally with the members of the audience. It's one of my favorite aspects of what I do. Often after a concert, I get a chance to talk to kids about Jesus, to pray with them, and to share with them how they can come to know the most important person in my life. (My husband Gary is the greatest guy on earth, but both he and I agree, Jesus is Number One in both of our lives.)

Almost every night, after the serious conversations are concluded, I talk "girl talk" with some of the young ladies at our concerts. It's always fun to hear about their dates, their new "loves," or their latest lament—how

totally "out of it" the guys are in their schools or
churches. We laugh a lot.

Frequently, the discussion comes around to me.
Someone may say, "I love your hair." Someone else may
comment, "I really like your outfit." Then there are the
"what about this or that?" questions and the "how do
you do?" questions, such as, "How do you stay in
shape?" or, "What can I do about my skin? It feels so
rough." You know, girl talk.

Usually my new friends are surprised to learn that I
am a lot like them, that I had some really lousy dates
along the way before I met Gary, or that there have been
times when I couldn't get my hair to do a thing! They
laugh when I tell them I've known that awful feeling in
the pit of my stomach, the one that comes when you
look in the mirror and see a humongous zit on your face
and Mr. Wonderful is picking you up in less than an
hour!

Speaking of zits, let's get one thing straight right
from the top. I don't like that term. I think it's
disgusting. If you want to use it, okay, but please don't
talk to me about z---. And plee-e-e-ze spare me the guys
who talk about "squeezing blackheads" and "popping
pimples" as though it were part of a religious experience.
How gross! Dermatologists generally describe those skin
blemishes as comedones or acne. That sounds better, but
a bit too formal for us.

Me? I call them "bumps." Isn't that much nicer?
Instead of a z-- or a pimple, you have a "bump." There.
Don't you feel better already? I just mention it here so
whenever I talk about "bumps" later in this book, you
won't get confused and start envisioning huge tumors
on your face.

Anyway, part of the reason I am writing this book is

*Name three qualities,
uniquely yours, that make
you different from anyone
else.*

We are not all knowledgeable in the same areas. That's why I asked Dana, Carter, and Joan for help on this book. Describe an area where you feel you are a budding expert. Now, think of something you'd like to do, but need help doing. Don't be ashamed to ask for help. The Bible says, "Where there is no guidance, the people fall, but in abundance of counselors there is victory"

(Proverbs 11:14).

that you keep asking me those questions . . . like, "What can I do about these bumps on my face?"

Two other factors make me feel sure that what I have to say will be helpful to you. First, I learned quite a bit about beauty, poise, confidence, and talent when I entered and won the Miss Florida Pageant and then placed in the top ten at the Miss America Pageant that same year.

Second, the scholarship money I received from the pageants enabled me to travel to Nashville and embark upon my career as a contemporary Christian singer. Since then, I have been privileged to work with a number of expert makeup artists, hairstylists, and fashion designers. I'll introduce you to some of them in this book.

For example, Dana Glover is a fashion model who is represented by one of the top modeling agencies in New York. She has appeared in dozens of well-known fashion magazines. Besides that, she is a dynamite saxophone player, a great singer, and a dedicated Christian. Dana performed as part of my band before moving to New York. She has contributed many of the beauty tips I will be sharing within these pages.

We'll also pick up some pointers from my friend Carter Bradley. Carter has done my makeup for most of my album covers. Among others, she makes up various female singers, including Taylor Dane, and the popular trio Exposé, and has done the makeup for several HBO comedy specials. Then there is Joan Tankersley. Joan is one of the most fun people I know. She has helped put together the "look" for some of the best known Christian artists in the world.

I've been thankful to have these three special ladies serving as consultants as I've worked on this book. I will give you a lot of practical tips, things that have worked for me and will probably work for you, but Dana, Carter, and Joan do this for a living. Their input, along with others to whom I will be referring, will give you that "professional edge."

All set? Okay, let's get started by looking in the mirror.

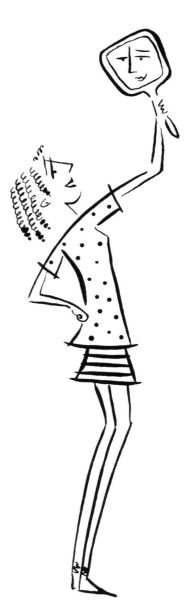

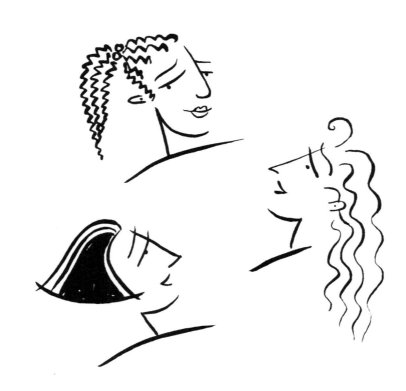

Face to Face

WHEN I WAS A LITTLE GIRL, MY MOM USED to tell me again and again, "Kim, take care of your skin. It's the only skin you get." Technically, Mom's warning was incorrect. Our skin cells are in a constant state of change: growing, dying, or reproducing. The dead cells on the surface of the body must be removed gently and replaced by new, living cells that have been developing beneath the surface, waiting patiently for their day to come.

Let no one ever come to you without coming away better and happier. Be the living expression of God's kindness: kindness in your face, kindness in your eyes, kindness in your smile, kindness in your warm greeting.

MOTHER TERESA

Nevertheless, the "spirit" of Mom's words was absolutely correct. Whatever you do to your skin, positively or negatively, you're going to have to live with for the rest of your life. Fortunately, bad skin can be improved, but it will take serious care and treatment. Apart from a miracle, no magic potions or late-night television "info-mercial" product (a product being hyped in "informative," thirty-minute commercials) is going to relieve you of your responsibility to take care of your own skin.

Your face is the primary medium through which other people get to know you. Your face expresses excitement, sadness, health, or sickness. I know it may be hard to imagine right now, but if you don't take good care of it, your face will someday be a billboard announcing that you are getting old before your time. Good skin care will not just make you more attractive now; it will prevent skin damage and help you to be prettier as you age.

In order to treat your skin properly, you need to be aware of some basic facts. Besides the obvious health and beauty benefits of understanding your skin, there are important financial ramifications as well. When it comes to skin care, what you don't know can hurt you. Ignorance of some simple truths will not only open you to potential skin damage, but it will also set you up to be ripped off. Let me explain.

I am constantly saddened to see teenage young women (and adult women, as well) who are being bilked by the beauty "experts" behind the cosmetics counters at their local department stores. Every woman wants to look a little better. Fine. But any cosmetics salesperson worth his or her fragrance knows that it's part of the job to convince you that you "need to do something about the way you look" rather than help you do better with what you have.

Keep in mind, Americans spend more than two and one half billion dollars every year on beauty products. (Some estimates go as high as sixteen billion per year!) Guess which part of that lucrative industry is growing the fastest. Yep, skin care products. So don't assume that the "expert" behind the counter has your best complexion in mind. More than likely, he or she is primarily interested in selling you some products.

While we're here, let's say a word about all those beautiful women and handsome hunks you see handing out sample products in your favorite department store. Don't ever allow yourself to forget (no matter how good looking that young sales guy is—and yes, more and more stores are using gorgeous guys to sell cosmetics to teenage girls) that nearly every employee you see in the cosmetics department is hoping to make a commission on what you buy. The moment you express even a passing interest in a product, you will be surrounded by a throng of salespeople. You may be momentarily flattered by all this doting, but believe me, these salespeople aren't trying to win your heart. They want to win your bucks.

Often, the salesperson who approaches you first is not even employed by the store. He or she works for the cosmetics company and has been specially trained in high-powered sales techniques. Since the more they sell, the more money they make, these salespersons are delighted to sell you their most expensive products, many of which you don't need, some of which may not be good for your face, and all of which are extremely overpriced.

When you purchase a product, what most determines your selection? Brand name? Quality? Price? Why?

SKIN CROSS SECTION

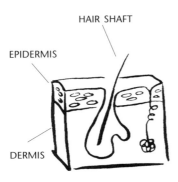

HAIR SHAFT

EPIDERMIS

DERMIS

A dear old Quaker lady, distinguished for her youthful appearance, was asked what she used to preserve her appearance. She replied sweetly, "I use for the lips, truth; for the voice, prayer; for the eyes, pity; for the hand, charity; for the figure, uprightness; and for the heart, love."

JERRY FLEISHMAN

WHAT YOU NEED TO KNOW ABOUT YOUR SKIN

Let's keep it simple. Basically your skin is comprised of two layers, the epidermis, which is the top, outer layer, and the dermis, the thick layer beneath the epidermis. The epidermis protects your lower levels of skin from the dangerous elements which constantly attack it: sun, cold, wind, bacteria, and other natural enemies, not to mention air pollution, acid rain, and a host of other man-made enemies. For the most part, the surface layer of the epidermis is made up of—I hate to tell you this— dead or dying cells.

But don't worry; you don't need to call your doctor, because as the outer layers of the epidermis die off, your body is busy manufacturing new cells just beneath the skin surface. As the new cells grow, they keep pushing toward the surface of your skin until they reach the outer levels. By that time, their life cycle is pretty much over, and they are either dead or rapidly dying themselves.

Nothing you do to your skin will bring these dead cells back to life again. The only thing to do with them is wash them away, cleansing your skin and making way for the new, younger generations of cells that are already pushing toward the top.

Naturally, this process is going on virtually unnoticed. The Lord designed your skin to perpetually reproduce itself, so about once a month, your old skin cells are replaced by new ones. Pretty amazing, isn't it?

While all the pushing, shoving, growing, and dying is happening in the epidermis, the dermis seems rather boring by comparison. But don't kid yourself; your dermis is definitely not dormant. In fact, this is the area of your skin where trouble often begins, and no wonder! The dermis contains oil, sweat glands, fat glands, hair follicles, blood vessels, nerves, and collagen, the substance that gives your skin its elastic qualities. Sounds like a bump waiting to happen, doesn't it?

Basically, most of the megabucks skin-care industry revolves around these two concerns:

1. Cleansing your skin of those dead layers of cells on your epidermis.
2. Preventing skin problems, many of which get their start in the dermis—problems such as blemishes, pimples, whiteheads, blackheads, other kinds of acne, scaling or flaking dry skin, chapping or chafing, lines and wrinkles, pigment changes, sagging skin, sun damage, sensitive skin, and others.

WOMAN: KNOW THY SKIN TYPE!

Although it is not one of God's commandments, it is certainly a rule that if you want to treat your skin accurately and adequately, you must determine what type of skin you have. You don't need to be a rocket scientist to figure it out, yet many young women slap all sorts of concoctions onto their faces without having a clue as to what the stuff is or what it will do to their type of skin. Just because a certain skin product works for your best friend is no guarantee it will help you at all. It could, in fact, harm your skin if it is not right for your skin type.

Skin types fall into three categories: dry, oily, and normal. It's really easy to understand these definitions.

Dry skin tends to dehydrate easily, causing flaking, sometimes itching, and often early wrinkling. People with pale complexions and fair hair frequently have dry skin. On the plus side, dry skin looks fabulous, especially in the younger years, if it is well cared for. If you have dry skin, you probably don't have many problems with pimples and other sorts of acne. Your biggest problem seems to be your friends with oily skin who all hate you

Let's face it, few women I know are satisfied with their markings, their height, their hair, teeth, or skin, or even their particular personalities! Coming to know God in Christ helps us to realize Someone loves us just the way we are. He likes our height, hair, and even our particular personality. . . . As you get to love Him who patterns you, you actually get to love and accept the pattern!

JILL BRISCOE
QUEEN OF HEARTS

Keep in mind that "normal" is a relative word. What is normal, anyhow? What is your definition of a "normal" teenager? What is your parents' definition of a "normal" teenager?

because your face never seems to break out as badly as their does.

The danger of dry skin is that it is extremely fragile. It burns easily in the sun, suffers badly in extreme temperatures, and tends to develop flaky patches. Then, too, don't forget about those premature wrinkling problems.

In the next chapter, I'll give you some tips to help care for all three types of skin, but first let's look at the other two types.

Oily skin is just that—oily. It has a shiny, greasy look and feel to it and is common with dark-haired, dark-skinned people. People with oily skin tend to have more problems with pimples, blackheads, and other forms of acne, especially near the nose and cheek areas. That's the bad news about oily skin.

The good news is that most oily skin improves with age. Oily skin is naturally lubricated, so it stays younger looking longer and is less likely to wrinkle and line than dry skin. Pimples, which are most prevalent during the teen years, begin to disappear, or at least become less of a problem, as the person with oily skin ages. As a result, your complexion will improve.

The term *normal* skin can be confusing. *Normal compared to what?* you may be wondering. Or worse, If I have dry skin or oily skin, am I abnormal?

In her book *The Beauty Principal*, actress Victoria Principal says, "The only people I know with normal skin are babies."[1]

I like to think of normal as the happy medium between dry skin and oily skin. It is the mid-range that we want to reach. Normal skin is moist, but not greasy; it is well lubricated but devoid of bumps or other blemishes. It has an attractive, rosy color (which indicates that the blood circulation in the lower levels is good) rather than a rough, irritated look and feel.

Understand, though, no two normal skins are exactly alike. Neither is there any certain amount of oil that your skin ought to be producing, nor dead cells that should be removed. As ambiguous as it sounds, the best thing we can say about normal skin is that it is balanced and healthy.

Many people have combination skin. Combination skin has areas of dryness (usually around the cheeks and eyes), as well as areas that are prone to oily patches, often in what is known as the T-zone—your forehead, nose, and chin. Skin-care professionals have differing opinions as to how to treat combination skin. Some feel that the separate areas of combination skin cannot all be treated the same. They suggest a separate regimen to care for each different area of your face. However, if this is not done correctly, your skin may look spotty. Sometimes it is difficult to know where one area ends and another begins. For instance, you may overmoisturize a dry area and have the oil spread out into an already oily part of your face. Guess what you get as a result. Uneven, muddy looking skin, possibly with increased acne.

Nearly ninety percent of modern women have a combination of dry and oily areas on their faces. That's why many skin-care professionals recommend treating the overall skin type properly, rather than attempting to deal with the separate zones of what most people call combination skin. For example, if you have dry skin, with only a few oily areas, don't worry about "spot treating" the oily areas, just use a regimen that cares for dry skin.

You will be better off if you simply do a good job of treating your predominant skin type. Nevertheless, if you are willing to expend the extra effort, spot treating may work for you.

There's something else important to keep in mind about skin types: they change. Almost all teenagers have oily skin at some point in their junior high and high school years, to one degree or another. At least eighty percent of today's teens report having problems with acne during their adolescent years. Don't panic. You and most of your friends will grow into adulthood and have various skin types. Some will have dry skin, and others will have oily skin. Some will have normal skin, and some will have combination skin. It all has to do with your glands and hormones.

Although we can't predict with certainty, here are some hints that will give you an idea of what to expect:

- If you rarely have a pimple and have never had to race out to buy a tube of over-the-counter acne medicine before facing your "public," you probably will have dry skin in the years ahead.
- If your skin is slightly greasy and you have occasional but moderate flare-ups of acne, most noticeably in the T-zone, you will probably have normal or combination skin.
- If your skin is extremely oily and you experience frequent and "violent" acne problems—we're talking bumps of biblical proportions—you will probably have oily skin as an adult. You may have some embarrassing moments now, but trust me, you will, most likely, have great skin by the time you hit your mid-twenties.

What area of your life causes you to feel most insecure? Is there anything you can do about it? Is it something you can change or a situation with which you must learn to live?

HOW TO DETERMINE YOUR SKIN TYPE

Are you still uncertain about your skin type? Try this simple test. All you need is a mild soap and some facial blotting paper. No blotting paper? Use a clean paper bag. Cut the paper into a minimum of four, one- to two-inch strips. Mark your four pieces of paper accordingly—one for your forehead, a second for your nose, a third for your chin, a fourth for your cheeks. The number and order is irrelevant.

Now, wash your face with lukewarm water and mild soap. Be sure to rinse your face thoroughly. Do not put any creams or moisturizers on your skin.

After about three hours (or the following morning if you do the procedure before bedtime), take the paper marked forehead and press it against your forehead for at least a slow count to ten. Don't rub it over the other areas of your face; just hold it against your forehead. Do the same for the other papers marked chin, nose, and cheeks. Now hold the papers up to a light and examine them. Where the papers are shiny, you have oily skin. Where the papers are dry or only slightly marked, you have dry skin. If your cheek areas show dry, but your forehead shows oil, you probably have combination skin. If your cheeks and your forehead are oily, your nose, chin, and the rest of your face probably have oily skin, too. Similarly, if all of your papers are clean, you can be fairly certain you have dry skin.

CARING FOR YOUR SKIN

Skin care should not be complicated or confusing, nor does it need to be a hassle. Actually, it can be quite enjoyable. By following a few simple steps and establishing some routine practices, keeping your skin looking great can be as easy as brushing your teeth.

Regardless of your skin type, the basic steps are pretty much the same: cleansing, toning, and moisturizing, in that order. The way you cleanse, tone,

As a ring of gold in a swine's snout, so is a beautiful woman who lacks discretion.

PROVERBS 11:22

I love this verse because it is so outrageous! The idea is: if we are careless about inner beauty, all our attempts at external adornments with skin-care products, makeup, pretty clothes, elaborate hairstyles, or fancy jewelry are like pinning a ring of gold on a pig's nose! God's Word gets right to the point, doesn't it?

and moisturize, and the skin-care products you use depend on what skin type you have. That's why it is so important that you know your skin type before trying various care regimens or products. We'll talk about caring for the individual types in the next few chapters, but first let me give you:

KIM'S COMMANDMENTS FOR BUYING SKIN-CARE PRODUCTS

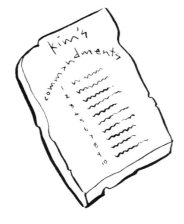

1. *Know your skin type.* I can't say it enough. If you're going shopping for skin-care products, don't leave home without knowing what type of skin you have. Buy only those products that match your type. For example, if you have dry skin, you will want products that help preserve the moisture in your skin. If you have oily skin, you certainly don't want to buy a product that is going to add oil; buy oil-free products instead. Nowadays, most products are marked for specific skin types.

2. *Become an avid label reader.* Don't let all the chemistry class names scare you. Check the labels for names such as collagen, elastin, aloe, and other natural proteins that keep your skin soft. Lanolin and mineral oils, although frequently used in skin-care products, may not be best for you, especially if you are breaking out a lot. Avoid them. They lie on top of your skin and aren't absorbed into it. As a result, your skin doesn't "breathe" as well, and you'll probably soon be breeding bumps.

3. *Go fragrance free.* Exotic-smelling ingredients may make the product more commercial, but usually they do no good for your skin. Also, the fragrance may irritate or otherwise negatively react with your skin.

4. *Check for preservatives.* Normally, these are the long,

tongue-twisting names of ingredients listed on the label. They are included in the product to keep it from spoiling. If a product doesn't have preservatives, that doesn't mean it's bad, merely that it will not have a long shelf life, so don't buy more than you need.

5. *Keep products coordinated.* Most manufacturers design their skin-care products to work in sync with each other. If you mix brands, you may not get the full effect you are hoping and paying for. Some products may even work against each other. Stick to the same brand unless you've discovered some secret formula that really works wonders for you.

6. *Don't be blinded by a pretty package.* The best product for your skin may not be the expensive, "designer" name brand. Prices for skin-care products can be out of sight, some as high as $75.00 an ounce! Don't be fooled. The most expensive products are not necessarily the best.

   Beware, too, those gorgeous sculpted glass bottles and beautifully decorated boxes. Unless you are a collector, most of them will end up in the trash. Regardless, the product in a plain plastic jar may be just as effective (and much less costly) than the one in the lovely container.

7. *Shop around.* As with most things associated with the health and beauty industries, prices for skin-care products vary widely. If you are shopping at Bloomingdale's, Neiman Marcus, or Saks Fifth Avenue, you are paying for ambiance, which is great, but does nothing for your skin. You may find similar products cheaper at your local discount drugstore.

8. *Buy small quantities.* Buy the smallest size if you have never used a particular product before. It is silly to

A joyful heart makes a cheerful face, but when the heart is sad, the spirit is broken.

PROVERBS 15:13

load up on something, no matter how super the price, until you know whether or not it will work for you.

9. *Give the products time to work.* Most companies suggest a minimum trial of three weeks, assuming regular usage. By then, your skin should have either a positive improvement or a negative reaction. If you feel any soreness or other irritations, immediately discontinue use of the product. No cosmetics company includes misery as part of its beauty regimen. If you have experienced a skin irritation and can't figure out the cause, check with a dermatologist before continuing use of any skin-care product.

10. *Be willing to change.* Your skin's condition is affected by all sorts of variables: climate, humidity, sun, diet, your body's metabolism, and of course, age. A product that worked for you when you were thirteen may not be best for you at eighteen years of age. Do you live in New York or Arizona? What about your ethnic background? Notice the skin changes other members of your family have experienced.

Certainly, physical factors such as getting sufficient sleep, eating a balanced diet, and drinking plenty of water will all affect your skin. Since your skin is in a constant state of change, it may require changes in the products you use or the habits you form if you want to keep it looking great.

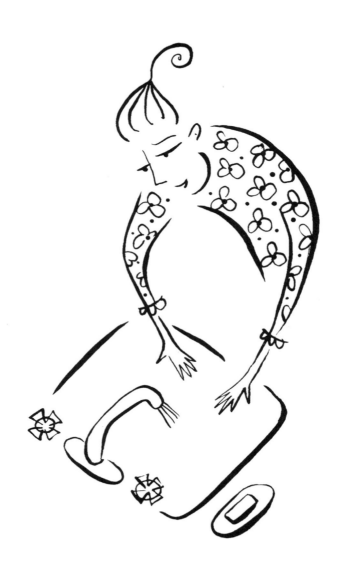

Three Simple Steps to Sensational Skin

IF YOU'RE LIKE ME, YOU MIGHT GET CONFUSED when you begin sorting through the plethora of books, videos, and skin-care products that are on the market. Surely, we think this skin-care thing must be a complicated matter. After all, how else could you explain all those health and beauty products? Really, though, a quality skin-care routine can be quite simple. The three main things to remember to do if you want your skin to stay soft and pretty, are cleanse, tone, and moisturize.

It's important to have a cleansing regimen for your skin; it's even more important to have a clean conscience and a clean heart.

For a good "spiritual cleansing regimen" look at King David's prayer in Psalm 51. (This is what he prayed after he had sinned by having sex with Bathsheba, a woman who was not his wife.)

STEP ONE: HOW CLEAN IS CLEAN?

By cleansing, I simply mean getting all the gunk off your face, including dirt, makeup, oil, perspiration, and all those dead cells I mentioned earlier. If you don't get all that stuff off your face daily, you will be a breakout waiting to happen.

Ideally, cleansing your facial skin is a twice-a-day job. Certainly, you will want to wash your face every morning, before you go to school or work. But for real cleansing, you will need a little extra time. If you can't do a thorough job each morning and evening, I suggest you establish a routine that can be done every night before you go to bed. No excuses, now. This is something you must get in the habit of doing, every night, no matter what. None of this "I'm too tired" or "I'll do twice as much tomorrow" or "Oh, I really didn't wear much makeup today; it won't matter." If you want good-looking skin, you've got to give it a thorough cleansing every night. Make it a rule: Never go to bed with makeup on your face!

You'd think that choosing a cleanser would be an uncomplicated matter, right? Well, think again. While everyone agrees that clean, fresh skin is the desired result, the suggested ways and means of getting there can be as diverse as the people you talk to or the advertisements you see.

Unfortunately, most problems created by improperly cared for skin begin right here, in the cleansing process. No group of skin-care products has more potential to irritate your skin than those designed for cleansing it.

The list of products to help you and me have cleaner, healthier skin seems endless: basic soaps, superfatted soaps, castile soaps (soaps that use olive oil rather than mineral oil as their base), deodorant soaps, facial soaps, detergent soaps, medicated soaps, cream cleansers, foam cleansers, cleansing gels, cleansing bars, nylon scrubs, cleansing milks, and exfoliating scrubs. Whew! And that's only a partial listing!

ALL SOAPS ARE NOT EQUAL

You might be thinking, "Aren't all soaps pretty much the same, with a few added ingredients here and there?" Nope, and those added ingredients can make a major difference in the way your face looks and feels. Some soaps are definitely more irritating than others. Here's a quick rundown that will help you decide which ones might be better for your skin.

Basic soap is the good, old-fashioned soap, the kind Grandma used to use. Basic soap is made from an alkali, a fat, some vegetable oil, and water. Plain soap and water is still the most common kind of cleanser, and it works! But it may not work as well for everybody. That's why the manufacturers add special ingredients to give their soaps "unique" qualities.

Superfatted soaps contain extra oils and fats. They do a great job of cleansing dry or normal skin, but because they leave an oily film, guess what they do for people with oily skin? Yep. Create acne.

Deodorant soaps contain chemicals to help fight bacteria on your skin, and if used regularly, are extremely effective at eliminating unpleasant odors caused by perspiration that has mixed with bacteria. Some of these soaps are mild enough to use on your face; most are not.

Acne soaps can be very valuable for a young woman with oily skin. These soaps are usually made without mineral oil, or at least they have less oil than other soaps. Obviously, for anyone fighting a battle against excessive oil on her face, any assistance is welcome. Still, don't

Many products will cleanse the dirt off your face, but only one can cleanse your heart—where true beauty starts.

The Bible says, "The blood of Jesus . . . cleanses us from all sin" (I John 1:7).

Have you ever wondered, "How can blood make me clean?"

expect miracles if your only anti-acne defense is a soap. Also, be aware that because these soaps use some heavy-duty cleansing agents, they can irritate your skin.

Detergent soaps sound as though you are buying something to clean windows with or to use in the washing machine. Most people assume that a detergent soap will be harsher than others, but such is not the case. Actually, some detergent soaps are less alkaline, less drying, and less irritating than plain soap. The advantage of using detergents in cleansing bars is that it is easier to control the pH balance. As a result, they are less irritating to your skin.

The pH scale measures whether something is acidic, alkaline, or neutral. The pH value of 7.0 is neutral. Anything higher is alkaline; anything lower is acidic. The pH of normal, healthy skin varies between 4.5 and 6.5.

So what's the big deal? Simply this: highly alkaline soaps may be too harsh for your skin and can strip it of its natural acidic quality. This can expose your epidermis to the elements and cause all sorts of irritations. On the other hand, if the pH factor in detergent soaps is balanced, they should be less irritating to your face. At least, that's the theory. Many familiar soaps, such as Dove (Lever Bros.), are really detergent bars.

Liquid cleansing products are being heavily hyped nowadays. Many of these products are designed for acne-prone skin or dry, sensitive skin. Actually, many liquid cleansing products are merely modified detergents in liquid form. If a detergent soap works for you, so will the liquid cleansers. Advertisers hype these products as being less irritating, but there is no tangible proof of that claim.

Specialty soaps such as aloe, vitamin E, and jojoba soaps are nice, but probably unnecessary. According to

Deborah Chase in *The New Medically Based No-Nonsense Beauty Book*, "Many dermatologists feel that soaps that are naturally designed to be less irritating achieve the same effects as soaps that have to rely on added anti-irritating properties."[1] Besides, most specialty soaps are extremely expensive.

Also, soaps with fruits, vegetables, or sweet-smelling herbs may have a pleasant scent, but they usually cost more and do virtually nothing to improve your skin. They also often have a high alcohol content which can irritate your skin.

Besides soap, all sorts of other cleansers are on the market today. Cold creams and cleansing creams are marketed as products that will clean your skin without stripping it of its natural oils. The impression is given in magazine and TV ads that any woman who really cares about her face would never use soap on it. Horror of horrors! Soap!

The great beautifier is a contented heart and a happy outlook.

GAYELORD HAUSER

What the advertisers don't tell you is that while most of these creams do dissolve the dirt and oils on the surface of the skin, the creams themselves leave behind an oily film that not only contains some of the dirt that the cream was supposed to remove, but will also be a convenient landing strip for new dirt. The truth is, your face will not get as clean with cold creams and other cleansing creams as it does with soap. Even the advertisers have figured this one out. Nowadays, we're hearing much more about products that "don't leave an oily film."

In all fairness, I must tell you that some water-soluble creams will do a good job of gently but thoroughly cleansing your face. But be sure the cream can be thoroughly rinsed off with water; otherwise you are just putting more dirt on your face.

In recent years, cleansing lotions and cleansing milks have also become popular. Many of the lotions have the same disadvantages as the creams, but some people with dry skin find them helpful. Milky cleansers are a combination of soap, water, mineral oil, and alcohol. They are usually quite effective for normal to oily skin.

WHAT'S BEST FOR ME?

My advice? Use an over-the-counter cleansing bar or liquid—with no fragrance or deodorant added—and water to cut through the grease and dirt on your face. Wet your face, and then apply cleanser to a washcloth. Spread it on your face and rub it thoroughly into your skin before rinsing with warm (but not hot) water. If you have dry skin, you may find that using a washcloth is too rough. If so, simply use your fingers to rub in the cleanser and rinse your face with handfuls of warm water. Pat your face dry with a clean towel, being careful not to rub your skin.

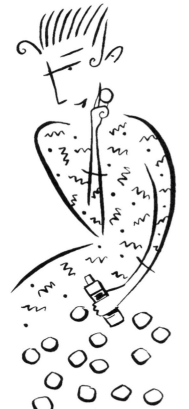

The basic principle for cleansing your skin is to use something that will remove the dirt but not dehydrate or add unnecessary oils to your skin. As to which type of cleanser you use, the decision is purely personal. What is important, however, is that the cleanser you use is consistent with your skin type. Once you have established that your skin is dry, normal, oily, or a combination, then choose your cleansing products accordingly.

REMOVING EYE MAKEUP

Eye-makeup removal is a bit of a trick. After all, most mascaras, shadows, and liners are made to resist water. If they weren't, when you go swimming or work up a sweat, your eye makeup would smear, run, and generally cause you to look like a creature from a B-grade horror movie! So be thankful for water-resistant eye makeup.

On the other hand, it takes some careful work to get the stuff off without irritating the extremely sensitive skin surrounding your eyes.

The best method is to use a non-oily remover made especially for that purpose. Soap and water alone won't do the job. Gently but thoroughly remove makeup according to the product's directions.

Do not use baby oil or petroleum jellies near your eyes. Oil does not dissolve in water. Unfortunately, many women have incurred severe eye problems as a result of smearing an oily product into their eyes. Others have endured blurred vision due to an oily film from their remover.

Eye makeup should be removed before you begin the general cleansing of your face to avoid rubbing mascara into the skin near your eyes.

STEP TWO: THE TONER TUNE-UP

In recent years, everything from clarifying agents and skin fresheners to astringents and toners has come to be known as toning lotion. The term toning lotion may be confusing because we think of "toning up" our muscles, so we think a toner must firm up the skin. But that is not what a skin toner does. A toning lotion is a liquid that is used to remove the last traces of grease and dirt from your face, residue that may have refused to budge despite your best cleansing efforts. It also removes any cleanser that was not rinsed away.

A toner is always used after you have cleansed your face, not before. You can't skip over step one, assuming, "If my toner is going to remove the last traces of dirt, I

Toners are used to remove that hard-to-reach grease and dirt out of your pores. Getting at those hard-to-budge areas of sin or negative habits in our lives is even more difficult.

In Matthew 23:25, 26, Jesus called a bunch of religious leaders hypocrites. He said, "You are so careful to polish the outside of the cup, but the inside is foul. . . . First cleanse the inside of the cup, and then the whole cup will be clean" (TLB).

Would Jesus say the same thing to you? Why or why not?

may as well let it do the cleansing work too." Don't even think about it. Toning products are not designed to work that way. Cleanse first, then tone.

Proper toning will refresh your skin, help close up your pores, and make your skin feel cool and invigorated. Nevertheless, because toners have astringent properties which remove the oil and dead cells from your skin, you should be careful what sort of toner you use. Again, most products are labeled according to the skin type for which they were designed.

Basically, toners can be divided into two types: those with alcohol and those without. Which should you use? Just remember that alcohol tends to dry the skin. Therefore, toner with a high level of alcohol may be helpful for someone with oily skin, but would be awful for someone with dry skin. The person with dry skin should use a toner that contains little or no alcohol. If you have normal skin, use a medium-strength toner.

Never use straight alcohol on your face as a skin toner. You could seriously damage your skin.

Use a clean, 100 percent cotton ball or pad when applying your toner. Avoid using other types of puffs and pads on your face. They frequently are made from wood fibers, which could scratch your skin.

By clearing away the last residue of makeup, dirt, or oil, you are making it easier for your moisturizer to be absorbed into your skin.

STEP THREE: MOISTURIZE YOUR SKIN!

The third step in your daily skin-care regimen is to moisturize your face. A moisturizer will seal in your skin's natural moisture and help replace lost moisture. As a result, your skin will look and feel softer.

It is important to understand that a moisturizer is

not intended to replace oil in your skin. Moisturizers don't lubricate your skin, but they do something equally important. They seal in the moisture that is already being produced by your skin. Believe it or not, it is the water in your skin that keeps it soft, not the oil.

Unfortunately for your face's sake, your skin's water easily evaporates, and if the supply is not replenished, your skin will feel tight, parched, and tough. Ordinary things you might encounter every day deplete your skin of its moisture: wind, sun, central heating or air conditioning, air pollution, perspiration, some soaps, and hot or cold weather. Also, if you fail to drink enough liquids, you will notice a difference in your face.

That's why I try to drink at least eight glasses of water every day. Besides flushing out my system, the water begins the process of moisturizing my skin from the inside, out.

I can almost hear you protesting, "Kim, you've got to be kidding! I could never drink eight glasses of water a day." Sure you can. Here's how I do it. First of all, notice I said I try to drink a lot of water every day. I don't get down on myself if I don't, but by a subtle shift in my habits, I've been able to drink more water and less soda and other less-healthy beverages.

For example, I drink water with all of my meals, usually instead of another beverage, and often in addition to whatever else I'm drinking. That's at least three glasses right there. Also, by drinking a glass of water before I eat a meal, I normally eat less, which helps me stay in shape. I usually have a glass of water when I wake up, so that's another. If I go past a water fountain in the mall or backstage at a concert, I usually stop to get a drink. When I take vitamins, I take them with water. Before you know it, I'm approaching my goal of

Jesus answered, "Everyone who drinks this water will be thirsty again, but whoever drinks the water I give him will never thirst. Indeed, the water I give him will become in him a spring of water welling up to eternal life."

JOHN 4:13, 14 (NIV)

eight glasses per day. Try it and see if you don't notice a real difference in the way your skin looks and feels.

The best moisturizers can't be bought at a department store beauty counter; they begin in your own body. God created your body to naturally moisturize your skin. Unfortunately, because of air pollution, sun damage, and other factors, most of us need as much help as we can get! Drink plenty of water, but don't avoid over-the-counter moisturizers. They can really make a difference in your skin.

WHAT IS A MOISTURIZER?

In your grandmother's day, women were limited to two basic kinds of moisturizing creams: cold cream and vanishing cream. Cold cream was the kind your grandma put on at night, or when nobody else could see her (especially Grandpa!), because cold creams were sticky, gooey, greasy, and gross, not to mention ugly. Vanishing creams were worn during the day and could be worn beneath a woman's makeup because the cream was less greasy. It "vanished." Unfortunately, they tended to make a woman's face look like a dull, flat, layer cake.

Believe it or not though, those vanishing creams were the ancestors of today's moisturizers. Today's moisturizers aren't greasy, however, and they don't make your skin look dull. Often, they can make your face look terrific!

Understand, it is impossible to moisturize your skin simply by soaking it with water. It will be wet, but not moisturized. Within a few minutes, the water will evaporate and your skin will feel dry again. To help prevent that evaporation, you must replace the skin's natural oils with another oil or occlusive (meaning, it won't allow the water to pass through) substance. The oil "traps" the water in

The essence of worldliness is the exclusion of God.

HENRY JACOBSEN

your skin, which is how cosmetic moisturizers work.

I suppose you could get the same effect by splashing your face with cool water for about five minutes, then quickly spreading a greasy substance such as Crisco onto your skin. Your skin cells would fill up with water and the grease would reduce evaporation. Granted, this method of moisturizing would cost you only a few pennies per day, but who wants to walk around with Crisco on her face all day . . . or all night?

Never fear. The cosmetics industry knows you don't want that greasy look, and they are prepared to help you with all kinds of moisturizers, which of course, will not cost a few pennies. They will cost dollars. Some cost big bucks. In some department stores, a two-ounce jar of moisturizer can cost $60 or more. Compare that to about $6 for an eight-ounce container of petrolatum-based moisturizer that you can probably find at your local drugstore. Also, keep in mind that these modern "miracle" creams are merely doing the same thing for you that your grandmother's cold creams and vanishing creams did for her (minus the grease or the pancake look). In other words, the old standbys such as petrolatum cost a lot less and will bring about the same results.

After cleansing and toning, your skin is much more ready to receive a fresh moisturizer. The same is true in our spiritual lives. When our hearts are calloused and covered with sin, we become hard women. But as the Lord strips away the layers of filth, our hard hearts become soft. At the same time, God's Spirit within us gives us a desire to walk with Him (see Ezekiel 36:25-29).

DO I REALLY NEED A MOISTURIZER?

Everyone's skin takes a beating from the environment. Consequently, most of us could benefit from a moisturizer. But the moisturizer required will vary with your skin type.

Most moisturizers are sold by weight. Oily skin, for example, needs a lightweight, oil-free moisturizer, and perhaps, if your skin is *very* oily, you may not need a moisturizer at all. Normal skin usually takes a medium-weight moisturizer, and if you have dry skin, use a heavier moisturizer. If you have combination skin, you may wish to use two separate moisturizing products.

Whatever weight you need, if you are going to spend the money to buy cosmetic moisturizers, look for ones that contain a bit of sun block, which will help protect you from regular sun exposure during the day (although these light sunscreens are not intended to protect against intense, prolonged, or direct sun, such as at the beach). Also look for ones that contain the chemical compounds urea and lactic acid, which will assist in cell renewal for night time use. As before, look for products that do not have a heavy oil base. You want to give your skin a drink, not plug it up with grease.

Before applying your moisturizer, wash your hands and face and apply toner. Be sure to leave your face damp. Remember, you are trying to seal in moisture. Now, put a small amount of moisturizer on your fingertips, and gently pat it onto your face and neck. You may want to use a special eye cream or throat cream, but it's not absolutely necessary.

Smooth the moisturizer gently. Don't pull at your skin. Never stretch your skin or press heavily on it. Facial skin and muscle tissue are delicate and should be treated tenderly. Treat your skin like fine, royal satin, because it is. After a little practice, you'll know when, where, and how to moisturize each part of your face. The main rule is: remember to moisturize.

Your skin is one of God's most ingenious creations. With just a little time and effort on your part, you can keep it looking sensational.

Mirrors show us the way we look, but what reflects the way we feel about ourselves?

GUARD YOUR LIFE-STYLE

Certainly, if soft, smooth skin is your goal, you need to look at your life-style. Going on a food binge, crash dieting, drinking alcoholic beverages, keeping too many late nights, and sun worshiping will all take a severe toll on your face. Smoking, too, is extremely harmful to your skin, as well as being destructive to your lungs.

Your diet has a great deal to do with the condition of your skin. Eileen Ford, founder of the famous Ford Model Agency agrees. In her *Book of Model Beauty*, she says:

> One reason our models have such good skin is because I have taught them to eat correctly. A poor diet will just about guarantee a poor complexion. Sweets, rich pastries, fried and oily foods, soft drinks, all may play havoc. A lack of protein or the right vegetables and a certain amount of fat can promote skin problems.[2]

Besides what you eat, what you drink also greatly affects your skin. One of the quickest ways to ruin your complexion is to drink alcoholic beverages. Certainly, there are plenty of other reasons to abstain from alcohol, but from a purely skin perspective, you should know that alcohol will dehydrate and coarsen even the finest skin in almost no time at all! It makes your skin feel dry and leathery. My advice? Avoid alcohol completely.

After food and drink (later we'll look more in depth at what foods are good and bad for your diet), one of the leading factors in the condition of your skin is the amount of sleep you get. If you continually shortchange yourself on sleep, your face will soon show it. I read about a woman who is in her sixties and is still considered one of the most beautiful women in the world. When asked about her beauty secret, she revealed

Other factors that can take a toll on your face are stress and worry. The Lord can help you deal with stress, and by trusting Him, you can alleviate worry, too.

Trust and worry are incompatible. You don't have to worry; God has promised that He will guide your steps. "Trust in the Lord with all your heart, and do not lean on your own understanding. In all your ways acknowledge Him, and He will make your paths straight" (Proverbs 3:5, 6).

that she never gets less than ten hours of sleep every night!

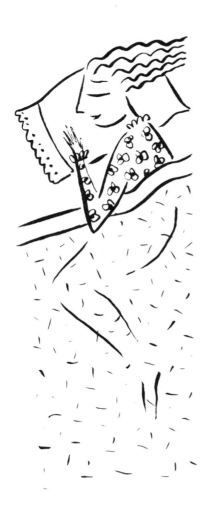

While ten hours a night may be an impossible dream for you (I know it is for me), sleep is one part of your internal and external beauty regimen that cannot be sacrificed without paying a high price. Sleep is the time when your entire body, including your skin, is revived. It is God's way of giving you a beauty bath every night.

Chelsea, a friend of mine who had gorgeous skin, began to develop a dull, pallid look. She also began to break out more frequently. When we talked about her life-style, she told me that she was averaging less than four hours of sleep a night. She was trying to compensate for her late hours by skipping church and sleeping away her Sundays. Not only did her skin condition deteriorate, but so did her spiritual health. When Chelsea adjusted her sleep habits, her complexion "miraculously" returned to its original beauty. She also started to attend church regularly again. That helped, too.

Another sure way to destroy your skin is to get too much sun. In a later chapter, we'll look more specifically at how sun can harm your skin and how you can avoid its harmful effects while still enjoying the great outdoors. For now, you should be aware that the deep, dark tan you've been working on all summer is slowly but surely turning your soft skin into leathery alligator scales. Don't do it!

Even the best skin-care system can't help you if you defeat its effects before they get started. On the other hand, if you are eating, drinking, and sleeping properly, while avoiding those practices that are harmful, your regimen of cleansing, toning, and moisturizing your skin will bring about marked, positive results.

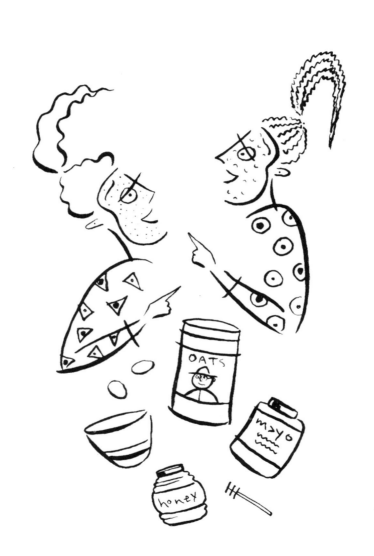

Maximum Masks, Fantastic Facials

BESIDES YOUR BASIC DAILY SKIN CARE program, once a week or so, just to be kind to yourself, give your skin some extra-special treatments. These could include a facial scrub, a facial mask, a home facial, or even a professional facial done by a skilled skin-care technician. These special treats will not only make your skin feel great, but they will also help keep your skin soft and clean. Here's a brief explanation of how they work.

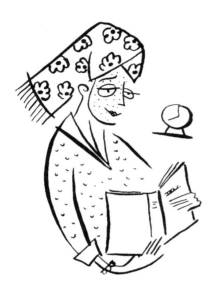

FACIAL SCRUBS

Advertisers tend to make most everything about your skin-care regimen sound more complicated than necessary. Nowhere is this more obvious than in the area of facial scrubs. Let's clear out the clutter.

A scrub is any product that has a mildly abrasive effect on your skin. For example, every time you use a washcloth on your face or a loofah (a rough, sponge-like cleaning tool) on your shoulders, you are using a type of scrub. A commercial facial scrub is usually a cream-based product containing tiny particles of a naturally abrasive substance that you smooth onto your face and then rinse off.

The scrub is just one more way to clean and remove the old, worn-out, dried-up, dead skin cells that are lying on the top layer of your skin. If the dead cells are not removed, your skin will look dull. The process by which these cells are removed is called exfoliation. As the top layers of dead cells are stripped off, the growth of new cells is stimulated in the lower levels of the epidermis. This growth gives your skin a fresh, clean, healthy look.

One word of caution. A scrub will not get rid of blemishes or acne. Never attempt to use a scrub as a means of scrubbing away pimples or other skin problems. In fact, you should not use a scrub on pimples or anywhere your skin may be irritated, cut, or broken.

Cosmetics companies will be happy to charge you plenty for facial scrubs. Although those scrubs are good, between you and me, you can make your own scrubs at home for just pennies. Try this: Mix one-quarter cup of regular oatmeal with a little water or plain yogurt. Make sure your fingers are clean before placing a bit of the mixture on your fingers and then gently smoothing it on your face. Steer clear of the area near your eyes. Now, massage the mixture into your face for a few minutes.

This is love: not that we loved God, but that he loved us and sent his Son as an atoning sacrifice for our sins.

I JOHN 4:10 (NIV)

Then rinse the mix off in warm water and follow with a toner and moisturizer.

If you've never tried a facial scrub, the idea of rubbing oatmeal and yogurt onto your face probably sounds ridiculous. Once you've tried it, however, your skin will never feel quite as clean without a scrub. You can also scrub other areas of your body in the same way. Your skin will look brighter and feel softer to the touch. Personally, if my schedule permits, I love to use a facial scrub three times per week. It's that good!

We are told to let our light shine, and if it does, we won't need to tell anybody it does. Lighthouses don't fire cannons to call attention to their shining—they just shine.
D. L. MOODY

FACIAL MASKS

Facial masks are one of the oldest cleansing products known to women, and still one of the most effective. There is probably no better way to give your skin an instant beauty boost than by using a facial mask.

What is a facial mask? Though the purposes of masks vary greatly—some moisturize, others stimulate, some exfoliate, and the most frequently used are probably those which deep cleanse—all masks work on the same principle. You mix up a concoction and smooth it onto your face. As it dries, the mask creates a mild tension and tightens your skin. After the mask is removed, your skin will feel incredibly soft and refreshed and have a wonderful, rosy look. Masks are fun to use and produce immediate results.

Most commercial cleansing masks can be divided into two categories: those that wash off and those that peel off. Wash-off masks are usually made from some form of clay or "mud" paste. After you apply the product to your face, the paste slowly dries, stimulating, tightening, and cleansing the skin as it does. As it hardens, it literally lifts excess dirt and oil off your face. The mask must then be removed with lukewarm water.

This sort of mask is especially good for a person with oily skin.

The second category of mask, the peel-off type, is applied to the face as a gel. Many of these masks are made with fruit, vegetables, or herbs and smell good enough to eat! As the gel dries, it looks like a sheet of sheer vinyl on your face. After it dries, it can be pulled off in large strips. Because the hardened gel does not absorb oil from the skin, it is good for dry or normal skin. When the mask comes off, it takes with it any loose, flaky, dry skin.

Masks work best when your skin is slightly warm and moist, and they should only be used after your face has been thoroughly cleansed. To apply the mask, put a little of the mixture on your clean fingertips, as you did with the scrub. Smooth it on your face, being careful to avoid your eyes. Then let it sit. After a few minutes, you'll feel it beginning to tighten your skin. Most masks are left on for fifteen to thirty minutes. During this time, don't plan on doing any heavy exertion. I also wouldn't advise visiting your bank. Granted, your mask will make you look rather strange for a few minutes, but once removed, it will help you look fabulously healthy a lot longer.

Don't use a mask too frequently, and don't leave one on your face too long. Furthermore, be extra careful when you remove a mask; if you are not cautious, you can seriously irritate your skin. Trish McEvoy, a skin-care specialist in New York City, warns, "More damage can be done to skin when removing a mask than when applying it. . . . Masks should be removed by splashing warm water onto the skin, then very gently going over the face once with a facecloth."[1] After you remove the mask, apply your favorite moisturizer.

As with many other health and beauty aids, you can

pay plenty of money for department store facial masks. On the other hand, for next to nothing you can enjoy the same benefits from ingredients you probably have in your cupboards or refrigerator. For example, a thin coating of plain yogurt or egg white is quite effective and brings a healthy glow to your skin. You may want to mix the egg whites and yogurt together and add a tablespoon of honey. This sort of mask is especially helpful for dry skin. Oatmeal masks are ideal for oily skin.

If you want to try mixing your own mask at home, here is a chart that provides the natural ingredients for masks that are appropriate to your skin type and the desired result. Remember, all of these ingredients must be mixed thoroughly before spreading them on your face. Also, be sure to avoid getting any of these materials near your eyes. The masks can be left on for twenty minutes and then removed easily with warm water. After rinsing, don't forget to moisturize.

Most everybody is looking for a good deal nowadays. Check out God's offer to you in Isaiah 55:1-3 where He invites those "who have no money" to come, buy, and eat.

MASKS FOR DRY SKIN*

BASIC:

1 egg yolk
1 pinch alum
1 teaspoon honey

STIMULATING:

1 egg yolk
1 teaspoon mayonnaise
1 drop mint extract
1 pinch alum

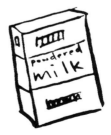

* From *The New Medically Based No-Nonsense Beauty Book* by Deborah Chase. Copyright © 1989 by Deborah Chase. Reprinted by permission of Henry Holt and Company, Inc.

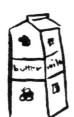

CELL RENEWAL:
1 tablespoon buttermilk
1 egg yolk
1/2 teaspoon honey
1 teaspoon mayonnaise

MASKS FOR NORMAL SKIN

BASIC:
1 egg white
1 teaspoon honey
1 teaspoon powdered skim milk
1 pinch alum

STIMULATING:
1 teaspoon Fuller's earth*
1 pinch alum
1 pinch baker's yeast
1 tablespoon distilled water

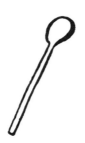

SOOTHING:
1 tablespoon ground oatmeal
2 tablespoons distilled water
1 teaspoon powdered milk

MASKS FOR OILY SKIN

BASIC:
1 tablespoon alcohol
1 tablespoon distilled water
1 tablespoon Fuller's earth*

STIMULATING:

1 tablespoon Fuller's earth*

1 pinch baker's yeast

1-1/2 tablespoons alcohol

1 pinch alum

SOOTHING:

1 tablespoon ground oatmeal

2 tablespoons skim milk

How can a clay mask get dirt out of your skin? Better still, how can red blood wash away our black sins and make our hearts whiter than snow? Pretty amazing, huh?

MASKS FOR ACNE-PRONE SKIN

BASIC:

2 teaspoons Fuller's earth*

1 tablespoon distilled water

1 pinch alum

1 drop mint extract

1 egg white

SOOTHING:

1 tablespoon ground oatmeal

1 tablespoon distilled water

1/2 tablespoon calamine lotion

MEDICATED:

1 egg white

1 tablespoon Fuller's earth*

1/4 teaspoon acne medication

* A clay-like substance that can be purchased at most cosmetics centers or drugstores.

Just as it is often beneficial to allow a specialist to treat your skin, it's also helpful to schedule a checkup with a spiritual counselor. Every so often, sit down with your pastor or youth pastor for a good heart-to-heart talk, not necessarily because something is wrong, but simply because you want to learn how to grow more Christlike.

HOME FACIALS

For a special treat, try giving yourself a home facial. It's easy, and it's fun. You could go out and buy an expensive portable steam machine, but why? Start by cleansing your face as usual, or give yourself a facial scrub for an extra-special treat. Then all you need to do is pour some very hot water into your bathroom sink and bend over the sink until your face is about two inches above the water. Drape a bath towel over your head and the sink to trap the steam. The steam will cause your pores to open.

After a few minutes, splash your face over and over with lukewarm water. This will flush out your pores. Then, slowly change the water to cool and continue splashing your face. This will cause your pores to close again. Now apply your favorite facial mask and relax for twenty or thirty minutes. Then rinse your face thoroughly and apply an astringent and moisturizer. Your face will feel smooth, soft, fresh, and incredibly clean!

You can also create your own "mini-facial sauna" by heating some water on the stove. Place the steaming water on a table and make a "tent" of your towel, stretching it over your head and the steaming water. Follow the same procedures as above. When you are done, splash on some cool water to close the pores, and moisturize your face. What a feeling!

PROFESSIONAL FACIALS

For the ultimate in facials and to give yourself an extra-special treat, try going to a skin-care specialist for a treatment. A licensed skin specialist will examine your face, deep cleanse your pores, remove any blackheads, give you a facial scrub, apply special masks, and give you a moisturizing treatment. Although such facials are expensive, you can probably learn enough from one or two visits to make it worth the money. Then once a week, or whenever you feel like it, you can give yourself a facial!

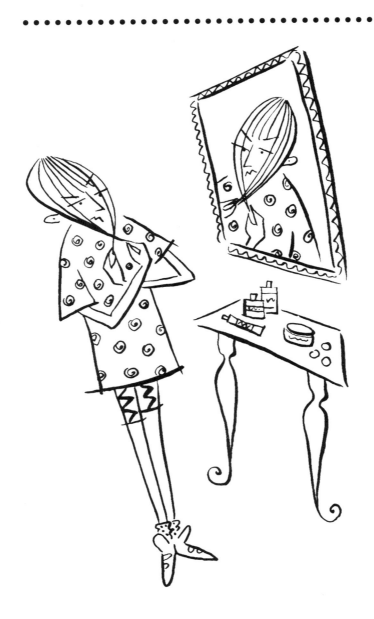

Breakout Breakthrough

WHAT CAUSES ACNE, ANYWAY? WHO GETS IT, and how can you control it? Actually, no one knows for sure what causes acne. All sorts of people have theories about acne's origins, but the underlying cause for acne has yet to be discovered.

When I need a reminder of how special I am to God, a passage of Scripture that really blows me away every time I read it is Psalm 139:13-18. It says that God made my body, that He knew all about me before I was even born, and that He is right here with me—right now. Check it out.

Dermatologists do have some suspicions, even though they can't pinpoint the cause specifically enough to cure or prevent those pesky pimples that pop out at the most inappropriate times. (Then again, I guess no time is really a good time for a pimple to appear.)

Perhaps the worst part about acne is what it does to your self-esteem. It's tough to feel good about the way you look when you know that you have this humongous thing sticking up on your nose. And that's the other painful part. No matter what the size or color variation of your acne, it always seems more noticeable to you than to anyone else—anyone, that is, except the class tease.

In every group, there's always somebody whose own self-image is going through the floorboards who feels duty bound to announce as loudly as possible, "Whoa! Nice zit on your forehead. What are ya growin' in that thing?" With friends like that. . . .

If it's any consolation, remember that acne is a common problem for eighty percent of today's teenagers. It plagues some people all of their lives.

WHAT CAUSES ACNE?

As I said, nobody knows for sure what causes acne, but dermatologists have a few hunches. They have also been able to sort out some of the things that for years were thought to cause acne, but don't. Some of these will surprise you.

For example, you don't get acne by eating chocolate, pizza, or fried foods. These foods may leave you looking like the Goodyear Blimp and will affect the overall appearance of your skin, but they don't seem to be the primary cause of acne. However, I do have a close friend who is convinced that every time she eats a piece of chocolate, it causes something awful to show up on her face. Who am I to argue with her? If you are certain that eating candy or French fries or whatever causes you to break out, don't eat candy or French fries or whatever. But for most people, eating candy or French fries is not the cause of their acne.

Another common misconception is that people who have acne must be dirty and don't have good personal hygiene, so their face breaks out. Not so. In fact, some people who wash their face several times each day may actually be their own worst enemies. They may be stimulating the oil glands in their skin to produce more oil than the skin can handle, which results in acne.

People often blame stress, tension, or emotional problems for acne. While it is true that these things seem to contribute to skin problems, again they are not the source.

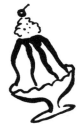

Basically, acne is created by overactive oil glands, which could be related to your diet, hormonal changes, or the genes you inherited from your parents. Though no one knows for certain what causes acne, for most modern teens all three factors are major contributors.

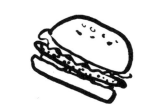

WHAT YOU EAT

Although most dermatologists agree that in the past diet has been greatly overrated as a cause of acne, most won't go so far as to say that pigging out on pizza, burgers, and fries will have no effect upon your skin. In fact, most dermatologists suggest that acne patients avoid these foods as well as sodas, citrus fruits, tomatoes, and shellfish such as shrimp, clams, and lobster. Apparently, too much iodide, a substance found in shellfish as well as in common table salt, can be bad for you if you are prone to acne.

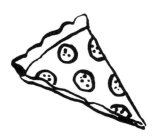

You should be aware that prescription drugs can also be a culprit when it comes to acne. Some people who rarely have a break-out problem begin to break out horribly while on medication. Of course, if medicine is the cause of your acne problem, the acne should disappear when you cease taking the prescription drug.

An old saying claims, "You are what you eat!" How could you apply the truth of that statement to your spiritual life?

BLAME IT ON YOUR HORMONES

Acne can often be caused by changes in your hormones. According to Dr. Michael Kalman, assistant professor of dermatology at Mt. Sinai School of Medicine in New York City, during puberty, your body produces an unusually large number of special hormones known as androgens.[1] This increased production is perfectly normal and is necessary for bone growth and the maturation of your sexual characteristics. Unfortunately, these hormones also stimulate your oil glands to produce too much oil. When that happens, out pops a pimple or a blackhead.

IT'S ALL IN THE GENES

You may be wondering, *Then why doesn't everybody in my class have zits?* Most do, at one time or another, but not everybody. A girl with dry skin, for example, usually has less of a problem with pimples, whiteheads, and blackheads simply because her skin is less oily. Don't get me wrong. People with dry skin still get bumps, just not as frequently or as severely as those with oily skin.

That's where heredity comes into play. If there is a history of acne in your family, chances are that you will have problems with acne outbreaks as well. Think of it as a family tradition. You can't change your genes; you can only learn to live with them.

BAD NEWS, GOOD NEWS

The bad news is that, at present, no cure for acne exists. Don't believe the advertisements that promise you quick relief if you will use their products. No product can keep you from getting bumps, and no known product will remove your acne problem once it appears. Remember, acne is not merely skin deep.

The good news is that we now have numerous prescription and over-the-counter products that can help us control acne.

TREATMENT OF ACNE

When it comes to complexion problems, control rather than cure is a realistic goal. Please don't try to powder or puff those bumps into oblivion, or try to hide them under layers of makeup or medicated creams. Extend your efforts toward clearing up your acne rather than covering it up.

It might help to understand a bit about how acne is formed. The sebaceous gland produces a substance known as sebum. We nonexperts simply refer to sebum as oil. If your face or hair is oily, you probably have very active sebaceous glands.

Both the skin on your face and your scalp have follicles out of which hair grows. Usually the oil on your scalp empties out of the follicle onto the hair and slides down the hair. The result, of course, is greasy hair. The follicle on your face, however, has only an undeveloped hair, so the oil tends to fill up and get stuck there. Acne forms whenever the follicle or skin pore gets plugged up by the oil or by dead skin cells. This results in either a blackhead, a whitehead, or a pimple, and although it gets pretty gross, let me explain the difference. Warning! This is not for those who are weak of stomach.

Nobody can make you feel inferior without your consent.

ELEANOR ROOSEVELT

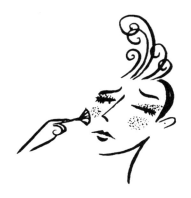

Blackheads are not pores filled with dirt; they are pores filled with oil. The trapped oil causes blackheads when the oil hardens, then turns black, or oxidizes, when exposed to the air. It's a simple chemical reaction. Honest! It has nothing to do with your face being dirty.

A whitehead forms when one of the many tiny hair follicles on your face becomes clogged with oil, causing a buildup of sebum that pushes to the surface of the skin. Pimples all start out as blackheads or whiteheads, and the culprit is the same: that nasty sebum stuff. When a pore gets blocked, it becomes a breeding ground for bacteria which feed on the oil trapped beneath the skin. The skin becomes irritated around the clogged area and may become inflamed or form a pus-fulled pimple. Pretty gross, huh?

Okay, enough technical information. The main thing you probably want to know is, "How can I get rid of those ugly, unwanted globs of oil?"

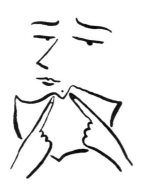

Start by washing your face with a mild soap and water. Then apply a hot towel or washcloth to your face to loosen the clogged-up oil. Before you gently press on the area around the pore, you'll want to cover your fingertips with a tissue so you don't spread any bacteria. If it is a blackhead you are extracting, keep pressing—gently—until you force out the hardened oil. Do not rub! It is also possible to remove a blackhead by using a comedone extractor, a pencil-like instrument with a tiny "donut" hole on its tip.

If it is a whitehead you wish to remove, the hot towel procedure is the same. Hold the hot cloth on the whitehead, then gently press on the skin around it. The sebum should come right out. Try not to break or tear the surrounding skin.

After the clogged oil is released, follow up by

repeatedly splashing the area, first with warm water, then with cool water. After you have dried your face, apply some antiseptic lotion on the treated area to enhance its healing.

Pimples should be treated similarly, applying hot towels to loosen the clogged sebum, but you must be patient with pimples. Here's the rule: remove no pimple before its time!

Many people make the mistake of attempting to squeeze or pick at pimples. Don't do it! Remember, although it is sebum that causes pimples as well as blackheads and whiteheads, if the pimple is not "mature," you won't be able to squeeze anything out of it. Furthermore, you may force the infected sebum out the bottom of the pore, thus spreading the infection even further. Picking at pimples may also cut or bruise the surrounding skin, leaving scars that sometimes last a lifetime.

Think of it this way, every time you touch a pimple with your fingers, you are probably spreading the infection. Keep your hands away from your face unless absolutely necessary.

In my family as I was growing up, we had a rule: "Don't pick bumps!" Our rule wasn't based so much on science as it was upon family tradition. The story goes that somebody somewhere hanging out in our family tree, picked and squeezed at a pimple and caused the infection to go backward until it eventually made its way to the brain and killed our relative. Now, please understand, this story may be totally fictitious, but it was enough to keep my sisters' and my fingers away from our faces!

We are unique. That means there is only one like us in the whole wide world. We have been handcrafted by the Divine Potter, stamped with the initials of the Master Designer. . . . We are made in His image, and He is unique. You can't help feeling special if you know you are the only one fashioned in such a way.

JILL BRISCOE
QUEEN OF HEARTS

If you can't be satisfied with what you have received, be thankful for what you have escaped.

EARL WILSON

Robert Schuller has said, "Beauty is mind-deep. You are as pretty—or as ugly— as you think you are. Think of yourself as a pleasant, friendly, cheerful, laughing, sparkling person, and your mind will make you into that kind of person."

Is that true? What determines or influences how you think about yourself? What do you think God thinks of you?

SCIENTIFIC BREAKTHROUGHS THAT REALLY CAN HELP

While my family folklore might not keep you from spreading infection on your face, today we have many medical advances in the treatment of acne that can help limit its spread. Many people attempt to control acne by drying out the skin with harsh soaps, alcohol, and drying lotions containing sulfur, resorcinol, or salicyclic acid. Sounds serious, doesn't it? Although these medicated soaps and lotions succeed in destroying the acne, they often can cause your skin to be red, rough, or chapped. The reason is that these are all peeling agents that remove the acne by removing the top layer of your skin. Ouch!

Doctors prefer to curb acne problems by prescribing antibiotics such as tetracycline, Accutane, and others. Again, these drugs are effective, but they also can cause side effects such as vaginal yeast infections. Check with your doctor before taking any medication, and be sure to ask about possible side effects. Doctors have at their disposal a number of new antibiotic lotions or gels that are highly effective at controlling serious cases of acne.

Of course, if your breakout problems are simply an occasional blackhead, whitehead, or pimple, your best bet is to stick to washing your face scrupulously every morning and every evening before bed, using a medicated lotion or an oil-free soap. Pat your face dry; never rub it vigorously or you may be turning small problems into bigger ones.

Try to remember, too, that breaking out is a normal part of life. Nobody enjoys bumps even in the best of times, let alone breakouts that occur at the worst possible moments. Still, keep in mind, most acne problems are temporary and will soon be part of your past. Surface bumps, like surface relationships, won't last.

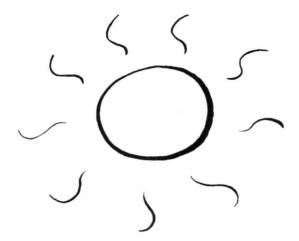

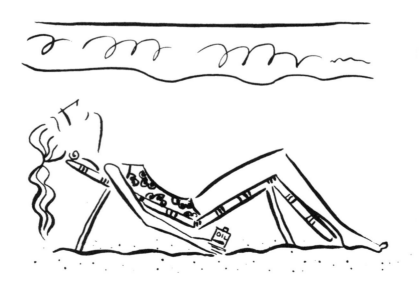

Say Good-Bye to Mr. Sunshine!

I WAS BORN AND RAISED IN THE HEART OF Florida, the Sunshine State. I was honored to represent our state at the Miss America Pageant in Atlantic City. So you can understand why it hurts me to tell you what I have to say next. If you want great-looking skin, and you want to avoid getting skin cancer, STAY OUT OF THE SUNSHINE! Unless, of course, you protect yourself by using a sunscreen with a sun protection factor (SPF) of 15 or higher.

I know, I know. As soon as the spring weather sets in, most of us can't wait to head for the beach, pool, or tanning booth. We've been duped into believing that a tanned body is a healthier body, and if your skin is pale, you must be sick. Actually, the exact opposite is true. A tan is really your body's way of trying to protect itself from the harmful rays of the sun.

Barely fifty years ago, suntans were considered to be "uncool." The only Caucasians with darkly tanned skin were mostly poor, "common laborers," who "unfortunately" had to work out in the sun. Pale skin was a sign of "class," prestige, luxury, and yes, even sex appeal. Nowadays, most of us have grown up with the idea that a beautiful body must be a tanned body.

While most everyone today agrees that a beautifully bronzed body is more attractive than a white, anemic-looking cast, few teenagers truly understand the damage that excessive sunbathing can cause. The truth is that exposing your skin to the sun is just about the absolute worst thing you can do to it. The sun is an enemy of your skin to be treated with caution, not a friend to be welcomed with open arms, an upturned face, and a semi-naked body. Sure, sure, the sun is an amazing creation of God, but so are mosquitoes. And yes, we do enjoy the sun's many benefits, including warmth, vitamin D, and other things, but that is still no excuse to destroy your skin by allowing the sun to fry it.

Sunshine will age your skin faster than anything. It is tough on all skin types. It makes oily skin oilier, irritates dry skin, and dries out normal skin. It robs your skin of valuable moisture, thus dehydrating it, and in many cases, it is the main cause of skin cancer. Although most types of skin cancer are not life threatening, there are some that are life threatening, and all can be disfiguring and extremely uncomfortable.

Overexposure to the sun means that the sun's powerful ultraviolet rays are not only browning your body, but they are also burning up your epidermis. Beyond that, ultraviolet (UV) rays can penetrate all the way down to your dermis. Remember that? The dermis is the layer of skin below the surface that contains your collagen and elastin fibers. These fibers are what give your skin a tight, good-looking, elastic quality, rather than a puffy, stretched-out, saggy, baggy look. When the sun's UV rays zap your collagen and destroy it, you can kiss your tight, taut skin good-bye.

Worse still, the sun's damage is cumulative and irreversible; it continues to build up over the years and it cannot be cured. A little burn this year, combined with the effects of a few burns last year, and the year before, and before you know it your skin is sixteen years old going on forty! Spots and wrinkles are certain to follow, and the "leather look" will be your legacy. No, not your clothes; I'm talking about your skin! Sure, it's cool to have a hot tan right now, but how hip will it be in a few years when your skin is as wrinkled as a raisin and your lovely face, lips, and body look like a lizard? If you think I'm exaggerating, take a good look at some middle-aged women you know who were sun worshipers in their teens and twenties. Look carefully at their faces and you will see spots, lines, and wrinkles that didn't have to be there, or might not have occurred until much later in life, if at all.

Don't get me wrong. I love the sun as much as you do. But when I found out some of the things I'm telling you, I decided that it wasn't worth it to slap on some tanning lotion, then lie out in the sun and get burned to a fried-chicken crisp.

Despite all the information concerning skin cancer, the pools and beaches are still packed with guys and girls who are frying their skin lobster red. Why do you think they do it?

I have extremely pale skin, so I need to be extra cautious in the sun. I'm an easy burn. But if I were thirteen years old again, I know one thing for certain. I wouldn't even think about going to the beach or pool without adequate sunscreen protection. As it is, even when I do spend time in the sun, I never allow my face to be unprotected. In fact, I haven't had my face in prolonged, direct sunlight since I was twenty years old, and I'm not going to tell you how many years ago that was! As a result of keeping my face out of the sun, my skin has stayed soft and healthy.

HELP AND HOPE FOR ADDICTED SUN WORSHIPERS

An interesting verse of Scripture says, "For I promise you: Because you have defiled my Temple with idols and evil sacrifices, therefore I will not spare you nor pity you at all" (Ezekiel 5:11, TLB). Have you ever considered your body as the temple of God's Holy Spirit? Could our sun worshiping be equated with a kind of idolatry?

Okay, so maybe it's unrealistic to think that you are going to stay inside with the window shutters closed up tight all summer. Even though you and I know that the safest way to protect your skin from the harmful effects of the sun is to stay out of it, we both know that probably isn't going to happen. Thankfully, for people like you (and me!), God allowed somebody to create sunscreens.

Sunscreens protect your skin from the sun's ultraviolet or UV rays. The sun emits three types of UV rays, classified simply as A, B, or C. UVC rays are short-wavelength rays which, for the most part, do not reach the earth. Most of them are absorbed by the earth's protective atmospheric shield known as the ozone layer. At present, sunscreen manufacturers concentrate on creating protection from UVA and UVB rays; they don't even worry about UVC rays. Unfortunately, with the continuing destruction of the ozone layer, due to humans' pollution, sunscreens may soon be necessary to avoid UVC ray burns as well.

Presently, UVA and UVB rays are most dangerous to your skin's health. Both types of rays can burn you. UVA rays do not cause as serious a sunburn as UVB rays, but in the long run, their effects may be more damaging. UVA rays can penetrate deeply into your dermis, producing long-term skin problems.

UVB rays, sometimes known by the misnomer the "tanning" rays, can also burn you. In fact, most common sunburns are because of overexposure to UVB rays.

If the sun is really putting out all that energy, how come we get so lazy when we sit out under it?

BILL VAUGHAN

SUNBURN, WHAT'S THE BIG DEAL?

Monica is a California girl who loves the beach. She has normal to oily skin, so she can stay in the sun much longer than I can, but she still burns. Despite all she knows about the dangers of sunburn, she remains indifferent to it. "So I burn," she says. "What's the big deal? I've been getting burned every year since I've been old enough to waddle down to the beach. First I burn, then I peel, then I turn brown for the rest of the summer. I always have one of the best tans on the beach. The guys love it, and that's all I care about."

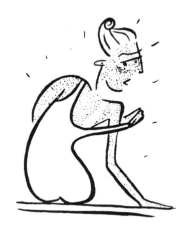

Silly girl. Monica may not realize it now, but she will eventually pay a high price for her indifference. It's like the old saying, "Pay me now, or pay me later." Payment is inevitable. Besides the pain and discomfort of her annual sunburn, there are a host of other problems the sun can create—premature aging, wrinkles, lines, sagging skin, and most serious of all, skin cancer. A good sunscreen could have prevented Monica's prognosis.

Even if you are one of those people who tans without burning, always remember that a tan is your body's way of trying to protect itself from the sun. The sun's harmful UVA rays cause your body to produce more melanin, a protein substance that darkens your skin. A gradual buildup of melanin, through shorter exposures to the sun over longer periods of time, will provide some protection from the sun's damaging rays. Still, the resulting tan is actually a thick layer of dead or dying skin, sort of a human suit of armor. Your best bet: use a sunscreen.

SELECTING A SUNSCREEN

There's a huge difference between mere suntan lotion or oil, and sunscreen or sunblock. Suntan products with no sunscreen offer you no protection at all against the sun's harmful rays. Sunscreens allow some of the rays to penetrate, making gradual tanning (as well as gradual burning) possible. A sunblock keeps out as many UV rays as possible, allowing you to be in the sun longer without burning.

Most of us consider the sun our "friend," and yet our friend can seriously hurt us. Do you have any other friends like that?

Sunscreens are rated by a number, their sun protection factor (SPF). This number indicates the amount of time you can stay out in the sunshine before you will begin to show signs of burning. Most SPF numbers range from two to fifteen, with a few that are higher. The higher the number, the more protection the sunscreen should afford from exposure to UVB rays.

Some people multiply the number of minutes they can safely stay in the sun without protection, times the number of their sunscreen, to estimate the time they can stay in the sun with protection. In other words, if you would ordinarily begin to burn after ten minutes, and you use a sunscreen with an SPF of ten, you should be able to stay in the sun one hundred minutes.

Keep in mind, however, that sunscreens are tested and rated under laboratory conditions without intense heat, humidity, wind, water, or altitude—factors that can greatly increase the damage the sun can do to your skin and decrease the effectiveness of your sunscreen. It is estimated that a sunscreen with an SPF rating of 15 in the lab could drop to a rating as low as 6 to 8 on the beach or at the pool.

Regardless of your skin type, and whether you tan easily or not, you should always use a sunscreen when you are sunbathing, or working or playing in direct sunlight. According to author Deborah Chase, "Doctors now feel that one should never use anything less than an SPF 15 sunscreen when going out into the sun."[1]

When choosing a sunscreen, look for a product with an SPF of at least 15 and one that contains PABA (para-aminobenzoic acid). PABA is a highly effective sunscreen (it may be listed on the label as Padimate O or Padimate A). You will still tan using a PABA sunscreen with an SPF of 15; it will take longer, but you will have less chance of seriously damaging your skin.

You should be aware, though, that some people cannot use products containing PABA. It may irritate their skin, sting their eyes, or cause some other adverse effect. It may also stain clothing. Consequently, many sunscreens are now using cinnanamates instead to block the UVB rays, and benzophenones and avobenzone to block the UVA rays. It all sounds very confusing, but if you are a beach lover or an outdoors person, it is well worth your time to educate yourself, and then look for these ingredients on the labels of your sunscreen products.

If you have dry or very light skin, look for an SPF rating of above 15. Granted, this sort of sunscreen will block out most of the sun's tanning rays, but at least you will be able to enjoy being outdoors with less fear of burning.

You can even purchase sunscreens that are

Inner beauty causes us to have a radiance that comes not from the sun, but from the Son—Jesus!

waterproof, although they tend to feel greasy and can block your pores, which can cause acne. If you have problems with bumps, be sure to pick waterproof sunscreens that are especially designed for oily skin. For further protection, you can even purchase sunscreens made especially for faces. Just be sure to buy according to your skin type. After all, if you are acne-prone, you certainly don't want to coat your face with a sunscreen loaded with oil.

When applying sun protection, don't forget about those sensitive areas such as your lips and nose. Zinc oxide, that old-fashioned white paste, is still one of the best coatings for these areas. Fortunately, the makers of zinc oxide have become more fashion conscious in recent years. Now, in addition to basic "lifeguard white," you can purchase the protective cream in neutral as well as all the colors of the rainbow and then some!

A Suntan without the Sun

If you love the look of a tan but don't want to risk being burned, you're in luck. Thanks to modern technology, you can now get a "suntan" without the sun.

Many fashion models today are using bronzing gels to give themselves a tanned look without ever spending time in the sun. Most gels last about three to four hours, which is great if you simply want to look good on a date. But don't forget Cinderella! Also, gels can be worn to the pool or beach because they are water-resistant. Nevertheless, keep in mind that gels provide only the look of a tan; they are no protection against the sun.

Another pseudo-tan can be achieved by using "quick tanning" products called self-tanners or self-tanning lotion. Most of these contain chemicals which react with your skin to produce a pigment in less than five hours.

The "quick tans" appear to be safe, as far as tests have revealed. At present, doctors are not totally sure, but they feel fairly certain that quick-tanning products do not damage the skin. Apparently they do not cause cancer. They do not produce allergic reactions. They can, however, produce bright orange skin (especially on your hands if you don't wash well after applying) and blotches if not evenly applied. Quick tans normally last about a week, then another application is required. Again, although you may look tan as a result of a "quick tan," you have not built up any actual protection in your skin. If you go into the sunshine, wear a sunscreen.

Tan accelerators have become popular recently. The idea is that by applying the product for several days before you head into the sunshine, you can get a darker, safer tan. So far, the "jury is still out" on the effectiveness of tan accelerators. About the only thing that has been proven so far is that they seem to be safe.

At least two "fake tans" are definitely suspect. "Suntan pills" have been declared unsafe by the U.S. Federal Food and Drug Administration (FDA).

Tanning booths have also received a negative reaction from dermatologists. Although most tanning machines use UVA rays, doctors are not thrilled with the idea of people purposely exposing themselves to radiation. Furthermore, they say that the booth timers allow too much exposure, and frequently the people using tanning beds and booths don't fully understand the risks. Again, until we get a definite "go" on tanning machines, I'd avoid them.

KIM'S TIPS FOR SUCCESSFUL SUNBATHING

If you must spend time if the sun, at least take these simple precautions:

1. Most importantly, apply a sunscreen at least thirty minutes prior to going out into the sun. It normally takes that long for the chemicals in most sunscreens to penetrate the top layer of your skin. If you go out before that time, or if you wait to put on your sunscreen after you are already in the sun, you will be unprotected for at least half an hour. If conditions are right, that is plenty of time in which to burn.

2. Don't scrimp on sunscreen. I know it is expensive, but so is damage to your skin. Sunscreen can be replaced; skin damage lasts a lifetime. Apply your sunscreen liberally.

3. Reapply your sunscreen frequently and at regular intervals. Apply sunscreen even if you are going into the water. The sun's rays reflect off the water and can burn any exposed areas of your skin. Moreover, sun passes through the water for several feet. That's why so many novice snorkelers get sunburned. They mistakenly believe that because they are beneath the water's surface, they are safe from sunburn. Many a vacation has been ruined that way.

4. Even if you are using a waterproof product, reapply your sunscreen when you come out of the water. Even good waterproof sunscreens will wear off after about an hour in the water. Be safe: reapply frequently.

The Old Testament provides an account of three guys who really took some heat but didn't get burned. Their story is in Daniel, chapter three. What was their secret?

5. You can burn at any time of the day, but the strongest UVB rays are between 10:00 a.m. and 2:00 p.m. Don't you have some shopping you could do during those times?

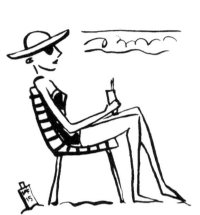

6. Cover your head and hair, and always wear sunglasses when in bright sunlight. Nowadays, sunglasses have become more of a fashion statement than a protection from the sun. Be cool in your shades if you want to be, but be certain that your sunglasses provide adequate protection against UV rays. The same UV rays that can damage your skin can also burn your hair and scalp and impair your vision.

7. Watch the temperature. Heat increases burn possibilities and so do humidity and wind. Water, too, causes your skin to burn easier.

8. Snowbunnies beware. Beach lovers aren't the only ones who need to take precautions against the sun. Believe it or not, you can "fry" your face on the ski slopes just as easily as on the beach. Any reflective surface such as snow, sand, or even cement can cause a burn. That's why it is possible to get a sunburn even while sitting under a beach umbrella. The sun reflecting off the sand is still potentially harmful.

9. Geography plays a part, too. The closer you are to the equator, the easier it is for the sun's rays to burn you. That is why you may never burn at home in New York or Chicago, but when you vacation in Florida, you get scorched.

10. Watch out for those lazy, hazy days. The sun does

not need to be visible in order for you to burn. Clouds are no match for powerful UV rays.

11. Attempt to tan slowly. At the first sign of pink skin or soreness, pack your bag and head for a cool shower. It takes several hours for the melanin to reach the surface of your skin, sometimes even two or three days! This is why you frequently find your skin tanning long after you are out of the sun. Unfortunately, if you remain in the sun until your skin begins changing colors, you damage your skin cells before the melanin can provide protection. The result? Sunburn, peeling, and flaking.

12. Don't go out in the sun if you are taking prescription drugs. The medicine may actually make it easier for you to burn.

13. Do not wear perfume if you are going into the sun. Your skin may blotch in areas where perfume has been applied.

14. Drink plenty of water when you are in the sun.

15. After sunbathing, take a long, lukewarm shower. Be sure to remove all oil, sweat, and suntan lotions. Pat your body dry; don't rub. Then liberally apply a body lotion and face cream.

IF YOU GET SUNBURNED

If, despite all my warnings, you still happen to get sunburned, whatever you do, don't put any oil on your burn. Have you ever seen oil poured into a hot frying pan? Something similar happens when you apply oil to hot skin. Yowee!

Instead, soak in a tub filled with cool water. Then try patting your burn with a soft washcloth dipped in apple cider vinegar. You'll smell a little funny, but it will take away the sting.

Here's another home remedy for sunburn: Put two cups of oatmeal (yes, oatmeal!) in a tub of lukewarm water, and soak in it for about twenty minutes. Afterward, wash gently with a mild soap. If possible, use a sheet rather than a towel to dry off; it won't rub as much. Apply an aloe sun relief product to the burned area. Of course, if you live near an aloe plant, you can simply whack off a piece of a leaf and rub it on the burn. Don't laugh. It works!

Oh, one more thing. As you are treating your sunburn, repeat after me, "I will never again go out in the sunshine without sunscreen." Say it again. "I will never . . ."

I don't believe in using my faith in Jesus Christ as a Band-Aid, naively thinking that if I do something silly or stupid (like staying out in the sun too long) that He is going to reverse the natural consequences of my actions. Still, it's good to know that even when I do something silly or stupid and get physically sick, He can heal my body. Aloe helps; doctors and hospitals help; but God does the healing.

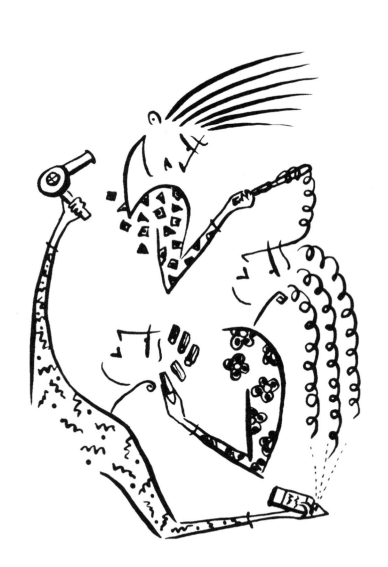

The Mane Event

TWO OF MY HUSBAND'S UNCLES ARE VERY successful hairstylists in the Pontiac, Michigan, area. Can you guess what inevitably causes them to want to duck under the counter? The customer who comes in waving a glamorous photograph of the hottest Hollywood star or the most recent pop phenom and saying, "I want my hair to look exactly like this!" My advice? Forget the impossible dream. Go with what God gave you and make the most of it.

The Bible says that a woman's hair is her glory (I Corinthians 11:15). It doesn't say that your hair needs to be thick or thin, blonde or brown, curled or straight, or look like a movie star's in order to top off your appearance.

Furthermore, no one type of hair is better or more desirable than another from a beauty perspective. Everyone knows that styles change like the wind. Throughout history, curly, straight, black, blonde, long, and short have all been the the rage at one time or another. If you think I'm joking, just look at the styles in your mom's high school yearbook photos.

HAIR CROSS SECTION

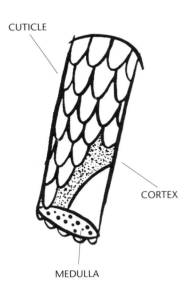

CUTICLE

CORTEX

MEDULLA

THE MASTER'S CUT

Your hair is made up of three layers: the cuticle, which is the outer protective layer; the cortex, the inner layer where the pigments that give your hair its color are produced; and the medulla, which scientists think (but aren't totally sure) gives your hair its strength and thickness. Admittedly, I don't spend too many evenings sitting around dreaming of my hair's cuticle, cortex, and medulla, but if you want your hair to look and feel great, you need to know a bit about all three areas.

Each strand of your hair grows out of a follicle in your scalp. The real growth takes place beneath the surface. Actually—and please don't get angry with me for telling you this—all the hair that you can see and feel on the top of your head, the stuff that you spend so much time, money, and energy combing, cutting, and conditioning . . . is already dead. Sorry! But like your skin, your hair is in a constant state of birth and maturation below the surface of your scalp. No matter how well or how poorly your hair is doing atop your head, it is only the hair beneath the scalp that is truly growing. The other stuff is just hanging in there. But we do want it to hang as nicely as possible!

The thickness or thinness of your hair has to do with its texture and color. Genetics determines the diameter and shape of each hair, which will determine whether your hair is thick or thin, curly or straight. It may surprise you, however, to learn that the number of hairs on your head is related to the color of your hair.

For example, blondes may not have more fun, but they do have more hair follicles, about 140,000 tiny, separate hairs. Redheads have the least, about 90,000, and brunettes fall somewhere in the middle of these two extremes. And to think that the Lord thinks you are so valuable, and He is so intimately interested in you, He has each of the hairs on your head numbered (Luke 12:6, 7)!

The average hair can grow six inches per year, and the usual hair life cycle is from two to six years. That means some of your hair can grow to be thirty-six inches long! Ordinarily, after the hair gets to a certain length, it seems to stop growing. When a hair reaches its maximum length, it lives a while longer, then falls out. Don't worry, it would be extremely rare for the many thousands of hairs on your head to all drop out at one time (although certain diseases do lead to eventual hair loss). Furthermore, the Lord designed your body so that about the time one hair is ready to fall out of the follicle, another is getting ready to pop up through.

If you coddle your hair and take exceptional care of it, you may forestall the inevitable fallout for a while, but take my word for it. Each hair will eventually fall out. Still, if heredity cooperates, and with plenty of pampering, hair can sometimes grow to incredibly long lengths. Country singer Crystal Gayle is a good example.

Have you ever wondered why the apostle Paul would refer to a woman's hair as her glory?

In Paul's day, women who were immoral often had shaved heads or very short hair. In contrast, long hair indicated a woman of virtue. Today, most of these stigmas have passed away, but we still equate certain "looks" with moral or immoral behavior. Can you think of a few?

The apostle Paul wrote: "Likewise, I want women to adorn themselves with proper clothing, modestly and discreetly, not with braided hair and gold or pearls or costly garments; but rather by means of good works, as befits women making a claim to godliness" (I Timothy 2:9, 10).

What's wrong with braiding your hair or wearing expensive things? Is that really Paul's point? What does this verse imply about inner beauty?

For years, Crystal's gorgeous hair has draped all the way down her back, nearly dragging on the floor! On her, it looks beautiful. On me? I think I'd have to go to a chiropractor to put my neck and back in place if I had that much hair.

While the amount of hair you have is related to its natural color, the type of hair you have probably corresponds to your skin type: oily, normal, or dry. In other words, if you have oily skin, most likely you will have oily hair. I'll give you some tips for each type as we go along, but no matter what type of hair you have, the basics of hair care are the same.

KIM'S "C-CRETS" TO SIMPLE HAIR CARE

KEEP IT CLEAN!

Regardless of the color, texture, style, or contour of your hair, the key to a great look is to keep your hair clean. Have you ever seen someone with dirty, greasy hair? Not a pretty sight, is it? No matter how hip, happening, cute, smart, athletic, or spiritual you are, dirty hair is a turn-off. Dirty hair doesn't win you many friends (or dates!). I have yet to hear a guy say, "Oh, wow! I just love Cindy's greasy hair." Sorry. It just doesn't happen.

On the other hand, I have heard plenty of comments (from girls and guys) such as "Denise's hair always looks so silky, soft, and shiny. I wonder how she does it?"

I can tell you one of her secrets. If Denise's hair looks good, it's because she is keeping it clean.

Something I can't tell you is how often you should wash your hair. Neither can the zillions of inane commercials on television that are sponsored by shampoo makers who want you to shampoo your hair once every two days, once a day, twice a day, or whenever you happen to see a red sports car. But you know when you need to shampoo, just by the look and feel of your hair.

If your scalp is itching, that is a pretty clear indicator that it's time for a washing. My hair is sort of dry, so I shampoo it once every two days. I used to wash it every day, but I noticed my hair was super dry and had a tendency to "fly away" on me. I asked my hairstylist about it, and he suggested that I wash it every other day. That one, simple step has worked wonders for my hair. On days between washings, I still rinse my hair thoroughly with warm water and use conditioner, which helps when I comb and style it, but I don't use shampoo on those days. If you have dry hair, try going shampoo-less for a day or two and see if it helps.

On the other hand, a person with oily hair will need to wash his or her hair more frequently than the person with dry hair. Still, it is not necessary to wash your hair every single day (although many women do). Be careful. You can wash your hair too frequently. Shampooing takes a toll on your hair. It strips the hair of moisture and oil, two essential ingredients for strong, shiny hair. Blow-drying and putting your hair in hot rollers also robs your hair of moisture. Be clean, but be careful you don't overdo it.

When you do shampoo, wet your hair thoroughly with warm water. Make sure your hair is completely soaked, not just damp. Then apply your shampoo. You don't need a lot; just a drop will do nicely. Massage the shampoo gently into your hair, rubbing it evenly throughout. Gently is the secret here. You don't need to rub, pound, or scrub as though you are trying to rid yourself of the memory of your old boyfriend. Take it easy. Let the shampoo do the work, not you.

We usually think of our hair as our "crown," to be kept clean and shiny. But in the Bible, Mary used her hair to wipe Jesus' feet (John 11:2)! What was she saying by this action?

Furthermore, if you have oily hair, your vigorous scrubbing may stimulate your scalp to produce even more excess oil. Use the tips of your fingers to massage your hair, but never scrape your scalp with your fingernails.

Let the lather remain on your hair for several minutes if possible. Then massage your scalp again before rinsing with warm water. Don't allow the water to "blast" your hair. This can damage or tangle your delicate wet hair. Just rinse smoothly and thoroughly. Ideally, you should rinse your hair for at least a minute, which is more than most people do. Try counting to sixty as you rinse. You'll notice that this is longer than you normally rinse, but it is more effective.

If you feel that your hair is still not its cleanest, you may want to shampoo again, the second time using half as much shampoo. Understand, though, once you have established a regular routine of hair care, "double dipping" your hair will probably not be necessary. The only people to benefit by your shampooing twice each time you wash your hair are the people who make and sell shampoo. Instead of shampooing twice, try washing your hair once with shampoo, then applying a conditioner (more on conditioners later).

When you are done, pat or blot your hair with a soft towel. Again, no wild rubbing. Be careful brushing your hair while it is wet. Wet hair stretches easily. It also pulls out of your head much easier than dry hair does, so treat it tenderly. Use a wide-toothed comb to get out any tangles.

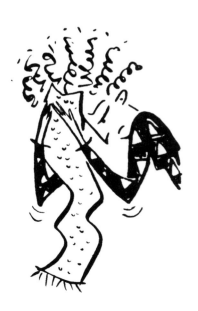

Speaking of combs and brushes: they can make or break your precious strands. Combing and brushing do more than merely shape your hair. They also stimulate the blood circulation of your scalp (though you should not scrape your scalp), which helps improve the life and health of your hair. Better brushes have natural (animal) bristles rather than nylon or other man-made materials. Your comb should be firm enough not to bend, with teeth that are evenly spaced but not too close together. Too fine a comb creates unnecessary strain when it is pulled through your hair.

Clean your combs and brushes often. Few things in life are more disgusting than a greasy, hair-clogged comb or brush. Besides that, dirty combs and brushes invite bacteria, which is then transferred to your head. You can clean your combs and brushes with the same shampoo you use, or for a more thorough job, add a tablespoon of your shampoo to a sink full of lukewarm water. Put in three drops of ammonia and swish your combs and brushes through the mixture. Then let them sit for ten or fifteen minutes before rinsing them with lots of lukewarm water. Be sure to dry the combs and brushes when you are done—no use asking for more bacteria.

When you comb or brush your hair, be careful not to yank and pull at it. Besides pulling hairs out, you can also break or split the ends of your hair if you comb or brush it roughly. Instead, use smooth, even strokes. If your hair is long, don't try to run the comb or brush from top to bottom in one stroke. Take only about six to eight inches at a time, holding each section with your free hand so you will cause the least amount of strain on your hair.

It really helps to brush your hair regularly, especially before washing it. Brushing removes some of the surface dirt and dust that get into your hair. It can also untangle your hair and move the oil along each strand more evenly. It is not necessary, however, to brush your hair one hundred strokes per day. Whoever came up with that rule should be shot by a hot blow dryer at sunup.

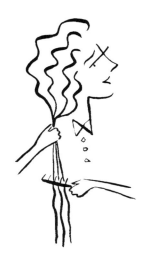

Absalom was a young man who really got hung up on his hair (II Samuel 18:9). What was his problem, anyway? Do you recognize any of Absalom's traits in yourself?

How to Choose Your Shampoo

The trick to discovering the shampoo that works best for you is balance. You want your shampoo to clean your hair thoroughly, stripping off the dirt and oil that make your hair look greasy, yet you want a product that will preserve, or even add, moisture and texture to your hair. Unfortunately, shampoo makers don't make your decision easy.

Shampoos are marketed for nearly every nuance of hair you can imagine. Advertisers encourage you to use separate shampoos for everything from split ends, to colored hair, to permed hair, and just about any combination in between. There are shampoos especially for short hair, long hair, limp hair, dull hair, damaged hair, you name it! It gets really confusing.

Fortunately, if you choose the wrong one, most shampoos will not damage your hair with normal use, unless you use a highly sulfuric dandruff shampoo on permed or colored hair. That could cause problems. More about that later.

The good news is that you can usually tell after only one washing whether or not a shampoo is good for you. If it leaves your hair shinier, softer, and easy to work with, hold onto it. If it makes your hair look limp, sticky, or dull, that shampoo is not your friend.

Basically, shampoos are of two types: 1) plain cleansing shampoos that do a great job of getting dirt out (but you will still need to use a conditioner), and 2) conditioning shampoos. Conditioning shampoos don't clean as well as cleansing shampoos, neither do they condition as well as special conditioners. But if you want your shampoo to do a little of both, a conditioning shampoo may be right for you. Many of today's shampoos fall into this category.

Under the two main headings, you will find

Choices are a constant part of life. How do you usually make your choices—with your head, your heart, or your purse?

shampoos with all sorts of extra ingredients, including moisturizers, oils and waxes, lemon (citric acid, actually; real lemon would rot), eggs (honest!), aloe, milk, medications to help control dandruff, balsam, birch, and even silk fibers to help your hair look shiny.

POUR ON THE CONDITIONER

Hair conditioners can be confusing, too. There are creme rinses, instant conditioners, deep-penetrating conditioners, bodybuilding conditioners, and products to repair damaged hair.

Creme rinses (also known as finishing rinses) were invented in the 1950s and are still one of the simplest ways of dealing with "flyaway" hair. These conditioners relax the hair and are especially effective with hair that is prone to tangling. They can help your hair to be bouncy and shiny, but they do not nourish it.

Instant conditioners are similar to creme rinses in that both are left on your hair for a few minutes, need to be rinsed out thoroughly, and are easy to use. They are quite helpful when applied to processed or damaged hair and can make other hair softer or less curly. There are instant conditioners available for all types of hair. Instant conditioners are more nourishing to your hair than creme rinses. They are effective detanglers and are especially good to use before swimming or going out in the sun to avoid discoloration of your hair.

Deep-penetrating conditioners are left on the hair from twenty to thirty minutes. They are thicker in substance and are great for dry or damaged hair. If you are going to have your hair colored or permed, it is a good idea to use a deep-penetrating conditioner a few days before processing your hair. Deep conditioning will help maintain moisture in your hair after it is processed

Keeping our hair soft and manageable is easy compared to keeping our hearts soft and sensitive to the Spirit of God. Think of some "spiritual softeners" that might be used for instant conditioning, deep conditioning, body-building, or structural repair.

and make it stronger and less brittle. Oily hair will probably not need deep conditioning.

Body builders are usually sold in individual packages and are designed to coat your hair and give it more body. Many of these products are effective but expensive.

Repair kits are conditioners that are actually absorbed by the hair; all of the others merely coat the strands of hair. These products are not to be rinsed out; they stay in your hair to help repair sun-damaged, brittle, colored, or over-permed hair. Again, they help, but at a high price.

Whatever conditioner you choose, be sure to wash your hair thoroughly before using it. Don't forget to rinse for at least a full minute to get out all the shampoo, dirt, and oil.

Apply the conditioner according to the instructions on the label. Most conditioners should be left in your hair at least one minute; some work best if left longer. When you are done, rinse the hair again; then wrap your head in a towel, patting your hair to dry it. Do not rub! This can cause unnecessary hair loss.

Carefully comb your hair with a wide-toothed comb and apply whatever styling or setting product you want to use. Your hair is ready to be styled.

When you have got a thing where you want it, it is a good thing to leave it where it is.
WINSTON CHURCHILL

CONTOURING YOUR HAIR

By contouring your hair, I mean styling and shaping it the way you want it to look after you have washed and conditioned it. In my grandmother's day, women used to sit for hours under hooded dryers at the "beauty shop" or under funny-looking drying bonnets at home in order to have their hair dried and set in place. (Believe it or not, those types of dryers are back in style today!) A hose usually connected the noisy, unsightly contraptions to the heat

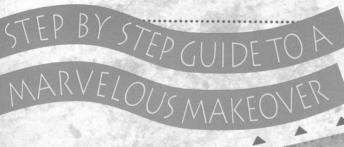

A STEP BY STEP GUIDE TO A MARVELOUS MAKEOVER

1. Always start with clean, moisturized skin.

2. Begin your makeup routine by plucking stray brow hairs. By doing this each day, you'll never need a major eyebrow tweezing session where you are more likely to over pluck brows.

3. Apply concealer under your eyes, on your eyelid, and to blemishes. Using a makeup sponge, blend concealer carefully.

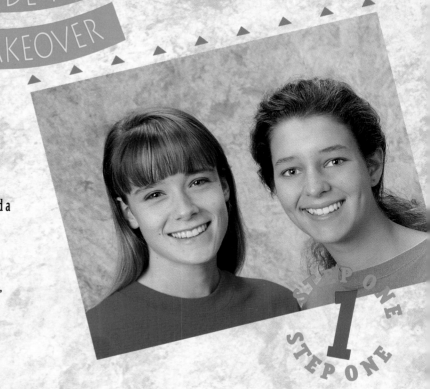

STEP ONE

4. **Foundation.** Using gentle strokes so your skin is not pulled excessively, apply a small amount of foundation to your face with your fingers. Blend foundation down onto your throat so there are no obvious color differences between facial skin and neck. Now use a makeup sponge to blend foundation around your hairline, nose, and chin to prevent obvious makeup lines.

5. **Powder.** Using the makeup sponge again, apply a small amount of loose, translucent powder to your entire face, including eyelids and throat. Again, use powder sparingly. Too much powder makes your face look chalky and wrinkled.

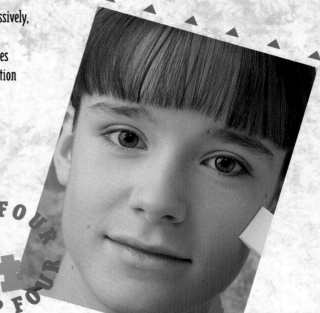

STEP FOUR

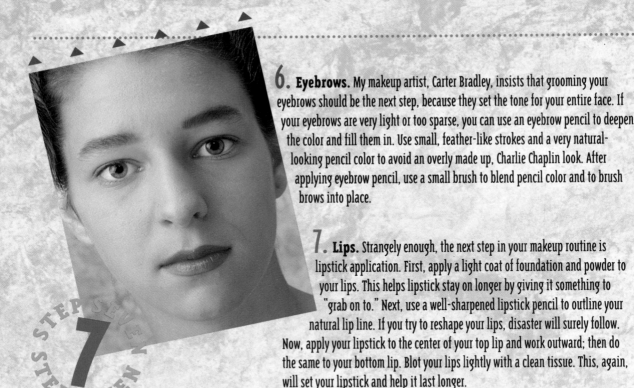

6. Eyebrows. My makeup artist, Carter Bradley, insists that grooming your eyebrows should be the next step, because they set the tone for your entire face. If your eyebrows are very light or too sparse, you can use an eyebrow pencil to deepen the color and fill them in. Use small, feather-like strokes and a very natural-looking pencil color to avoid an overly made up, Charlie Chaplin look. After applying eyebrow pencil, use a small brush to blend pencil color and to brush brows into place.

7. Lips. Strangely enough, the next step in your makeup routine is lipstick application. First, apply a light coat of foundation and powder to your lips. This helps lipstick stay on longer by giving it something to "grab on to." Next, use a well-sharpened lipstick pencil to outline your natural lip line. If you try to reshape your lips, disaster will surely follow. Now, apply your lipstick to the center of your top lip and work outward; then do the same to your bottom lip. Blot your lips lightly with a clean tissue. This, again, will set your lipstick and help it last longer.

STEP SEVEN
7

8. Eyeshadow. There are three different areas surrounding the eye—eyelid, crease, and brow bone—so we use three shades of eyeshadow. Apply the lightest shade to your brow bone, from just under your eyebrow down to the crease of your eye. Next, apply the deepest shade to the crease of your eye by following the crease from the inside corner of your eye to the outside corner. At the outside corner of your eye, bring a bit of this shadow down onto the corner of your eye. Now apply the medium shade of eyeshadow to your eyelid. Cover your entire eyelid and blend a bit of this color into the deepest shade in the crease of your eye to prevent definite color lines between eyeshadows.

STEP EIGHT
8
STEP EIGH

9. **Eyeliner.** For daytime makeup, you may want to skip this step or just apply a fine line of the deepest eyeshadow color underneath the outside of your lower lashes. If you do want to apply eyeliner, use an eyeliner pencil to apply a very fine pencil line as close to the eyelashes as possible from the inner corner of your eye outward. Smudge the pencil line with a pointed sponge applicator or cotton swab.

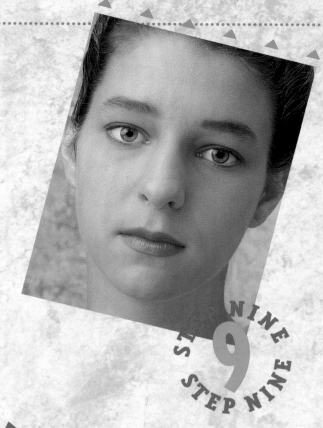

STEP NINE
9
STEP NINE

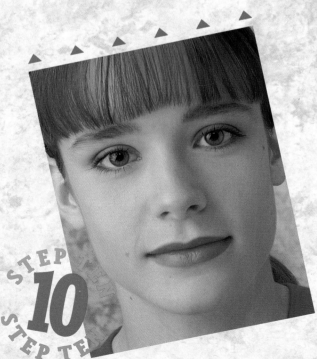

STEP
10
STEP TEN

10. **Eyelashes.** For the lushest lashes possible, begin by using an eyelash curler. Hold it on your lashes for five to ten seconds, then apply a thin coat of mascara. Allow mascara to dry completely, and then, using a small comb made for eyelashes, gently comb through your lashes to separate them. Apply another thin coat of mascara.

11. **Blush.** Using a medium-sized makeup brush, apply blush to the lower half of your cheekbone. Be sure to apply blush sparingly. Don't apply blush to the cheekbone area within approximately two inches on either side of your nose. This will prevent the blush from looking too heavy and unnatural.

12. Use a makeup sponge to blend in blush and foundation once again. Remember, the key to the most natural-looking makeup is to apply all colors sparingly and blend well.

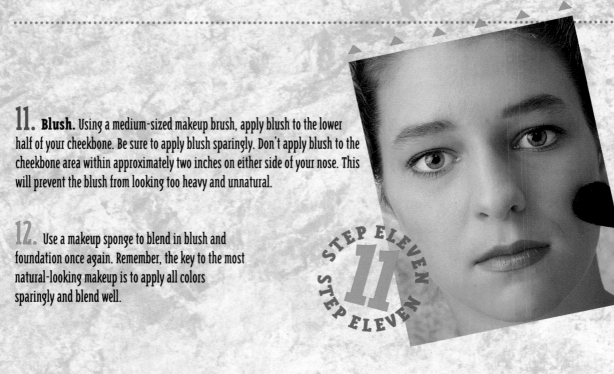

STEP ELEVEN
STEP ELEVEN
11

DONE!–and YOU look fantastic!

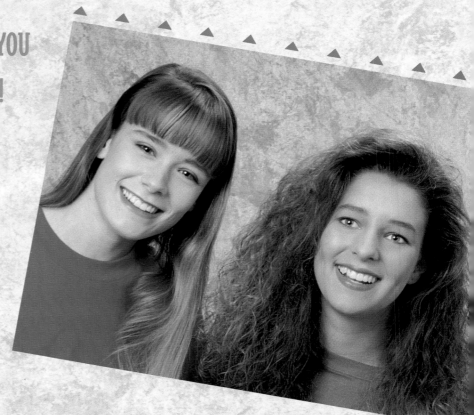

source, and Grandma would waste away the lonely hours by reading or trying to talk louder than the mayhem to the woman sitting next to her. Thankfully, today we have hand-held blow dryers, electric rollers, and curling irons.

BLOW DRYERS

For most of us, a blow dryer is a must. Blow-drying is a quick, easy way for women (and men) on the go to get going and stop spending so much time drying and styling their hair. Blow-drying, however, can be extremely hard on your hair, especially if you blow-dry it every day. Over-drying can make your hair brittle and frizzy, and leave you with split ends. Here are a few things to keep in mind.

Don't be overpowered when selecting your dryer. You don't need a blowtorch; you just want a blow dryer. Dryers now can be purchased with 1500 watts of power and more. These dryers deliver hot air with temperatures as high as a scorching 160 degrees. That kind of heat can really damage your hair if you aren't careful.

Also, choose a lightweight blow dryer. Some dryers are so heavy you feel as though you are lugging around a machine gun. Unless you plan to use your dryer as a free weight to work out your arms, go for something lighter. Besides, when your dryer is too heavy, you are tempted to try to dry your hair quicker, just so you can put your arms down! This often results in burning your hair.

I'd also suggest skipping all those weight-adding, fancy attachments, other than a diffuser. A diffuser fits on the end of your dryer and helps distribute the heat more evenly. It keeps your curls curly while it prevents blasting your hair.

Here are some other helpful hints for blow-drying your hair:

Blow dryers help us speed up the hair-drying process, but when it comes to your inner life, some things can't be rushed. Things like growth and maturity take time, work, and energy. Don't get discouraged if you feel your progress is slow; just keep moving in the Lord's direction.

When someone compliments you on your hair, how do you usually respond? What is the difference between self-worth and self-worship?

1. Keep the dryer on a lower heat setting, if possible. Often, if you allow your hair to air dry for a few minutes before blow drying, you won't need as much heat to get it dry.

2. Always hold the dryer at least six inches away from your head. I know; I know. Your hair dries more quickly when you stick that blowtorch right into the middle of your mane, but you are damaging your hair every time you do that. I have discovered that when I am in a hurry, I am tempted to allow my dryer to creep closer to my head, so I try to allow myself more time for drying.

3. Keep the dryer moving. Don't get so absorbed by that new song on your radio or cassette player that you absentmindedly hold the dryer too long in one spot.

4. Remember, always pat your hair dry before blow-drying. Never try to blow-dry soaking-wet hair; it will take too long, but more importantly, you will be exposing your hair to an extremely long session of hot-air blasting. Besides that, your arms will feel like rubber bands before you are done.

5. Begin drying at the back of your hair. Do underneath first, then move to the top and sides. Remember, don't pull your brush roughly through your hair. Use even, smooth, and gentle strokes.

6. Use a "vent" brush, one that allows the air to blow through the brush as it dries.

7. Some stylists suggest dividing your hair into four sections before you begin—back, right side, left side, and top (or crown). Use hair clips to keep the other three sections out of the way while you are working on one.

8. Whether you clip or not, when blow-drying, gently

twirl your brush under a small section of your hair. Don't try to grab a huge glob of hair, just a tiny bit. Dry that section, keeping the blow dryer moving all around the hair. Work from the roots of your hair outward toward the ends. Then move to the next section.

9. For more fullness, especially for longer hair, bend over and dry your hair toward the floor. Then when your hair is nearly dry, but not completely, flip your head back to an upright position and continue styling. You will be delighted at the added fullness to your hair. For even extra fullness, especially for a tousled look, try "scrunching." This is done when your hair is almost completely dry. Apply some mousse or gel to your hair. Pick up a small section of hair, and with a lifting and squeezing motion, continue to dry your hair. The diffuser attachment to your hair dryer is especially helpful for this type of style. The diffuser prevents your scrunched curls from being straightened. Work around your head until all the hair has been scrunched.

10. When you are almost done styling your hair, turn the dryer to a cool setting. This helps to dry any perspiration on your head and forehead. This is one little trick that will help your style hold much longer.

HOT ROLLERS

Hot rollers are a fabulous means of creating soft bouncy curls in your hair. Again, in the old days, women used to sleep on pointed or lumpy rollers all night, or they would hang around the house with their hair up in rollers half the day in order to get the same effect you and I can get in ten or fifteen minutes using hot rollers.

Consider your hair type before you buy rollers,

though. Is your hair thick, fine, tinted, naturally curly, dry, or oily? Various hair types require different types of rollers. For example, a hot-mist roller is excellent for dry or processed hair. Oily hair, however, will not hold as well using hot-mist rollers. As always, read the instructions or label before buying.

Generally, the bigger the roller, the looser the curl you will create. The longer you leave the rollers in your hair, the tighter the curl will be.

Here are a few more tips for incredible curls:

1. Use end papers whenever possible to prevent split ends. End papers are tiny, thin, rectangular papers that you can purchase at most drugstores or styling salons (as a less-expensive alternative you could also use toilet tissue). Fold these papers over the ends of your hair before using hot rollers. This helps protect the ends from the rollers' heat while also creating straight-ended, even curls.

2. Hot rollers work best when you have just washed and thoroughly dried your hair.

3. When you roll your hair, do it in the direction you want the curls to go—under, up, or whatever. For more curl, use more rollers of a smaller size.

4. The length of your hair and how much curl you want will determine how long you need to leave in the rollers. Longer hair needs to be in rollers longer. If you only want a light curl, don't leave the rollers in as long. Otherwise, make sure the rollers are completely cool before you take them out. If you take the rollers out too soon, the curl won't last.

5. When you remove the rollers, start at the back of your neck and work upward. Don't pull or your hair will be a tangled mess.

6. After the rollers are out, let the curls cool a bit longer before brushing. Your set will last longer.

COLD CURLERS

If you don't mind rollers in your hair for long periods of time, soft sponge rollers are much more gentle on your locks than hot rollers. You can even sleep on them without damaging your hair. The disadvantage is obvious: letting your hair dry naturally with cold rollers in it takes much more time than curling it with hot rollers. If your immediate appearance is important, cold curlers will cause you to want to put a paper bag over your head. We've all heard the jokes from guys who have seen us in rollers. "Hey, how many channels can you get on those things?" In other words, if you need to be somewhere, looking good, soon, I'd skip the cold rollers. Or, if that special guy will be over in twenty-five minutes, forget cold rollers and reach for a blow dryer or hot rollers.

CURLING IRONS

Curling irons are great for that special twist, wave, or curl you want to put in at just the right place They are also good for quick touch-ups on your hair. Unfortunately, curling irons can also burn or damage your hair easier and more quickly than any other styling tool. If you use a curling iron, you must use it carefully and correctly.

Curling irons come in several sizes. The size of the rod, which extends from the handle, determines the size of the curl. Before you purchase an iron and experiment on your own, I'd advise you to have a professional hair-stylist show you how to use a curling iron correctly. It is that delicate of a procedure. Think of it as ironing your hair. You can destroy your clothing by holding a hot iron in one place too long or leaving it at too high a temperature, and you can do the same thing to your hair.

Don't get me wrong. A curling iron can help you create sensational curls—I wouldn't go on a trip without mine—but you need to be extremely careful when using one. Here are some tips:

1. Make sure your hair is dry before you attempt to use a curling iron. Never use a curling iron on wet hair!

2. Don't keep the iron on your hair for long. Hair that took you months to grow can break in seconds when you are using a curling iron.

3. Curl only a small section of hair at a time. If you want more curl, use rollers.

4. Never let the wand touch your scalp. And although it may seem obvious, I have seen enough young women with burns caused by curling irons that I'm going to remind you anyway. Never touch the styling wand itself with your fingers! Also, keep the curling iron away from water. Especially dangerous are wet sinks or vanity countertops.

5. How does a curling iron work? The curls are created by tucking the hair into the iron's crimper and rolling your hair around the iron. Most irons have a spring mechanism to help hold the hair in place while you are curling it. But don't keep your hair in the crimper too long, unless you're going for that "damaged hair" look!

Whether you use a blow dryer, hot rollers, a curling iron, or a combination of the three, keep in mind that heat is no help to your hair. To counteract the effects of hot styling, condition your hair regularly. Also, whenever possible, give your hair a break and let it dry naturally. Applying a styling lotion, mousse, or gel to your hair before drying can also help prevent heat damage.

God loves each of us as if there were only one of us.
AUGUSTINE

STICKY STYLING PRODUCTS

The other day I was looking at a photo of myself taken in 1984 at the Miss Florida Pageant. What I noticed was not my gown, or my figure, or my skin. My attention was riveted to my hair. It was much longer than I wear it now, and the stylist who cut it did a wonderful job for me. Still, I was struck by how "stuck together" every strand of hair looked. Then I remembered. Back then the goal was to get your hair to stay in one place for the longest period of time possible. Any styling product short of cement that helped do that was considered a blessing.

Today we want our hairstyles to look and feel "natural" and to move with our bodies. Some highly stylized "dos" that are shown in magazines are great for photographs, fashion layouts, and special occasions, but they are definitley not for everyday wear. The helmet-head look is definitely out, hopefully for good. Thankfully, we now have a number of choices to help our hair stay put without making it look as though we are wearing protective headgear. We have setting lotions, mousses, gels, and less-stifling hair sprays. Here's a quick rundown on what you need to know about them:

- *Setting lotions* are used on your hair after it has been washed but while it is still wet. Then the hair is placed in rollers or clips. As the hair dries, the lotion coats the hair, prolonging the style.
- *Mousses* are foams that can be applied to damp, freshly washed hair. Mousses work especially well when you blow-dry your hair.
- *Gels* are clear, thick products used, again, on damp, freshly washed hair. They are great for creating a slick, wet look, while holding the hair stiffly in one place. They are also good for unusual styles that seem to defy gravity. Spray-on gels accomplish the same results without being as stiff or wet-looking as regular gels.

Two problems surround the above style setters. First, because many setting lotions, mousses, and gels have a high alcohol content, they can be extremely drying to your hair, perhaps too drying for damaged, permed, colored, or naturally dry hair. If dryness is a problem for you, look for alcohol-free products. Second, many of these setting products cause your hair to be sticky, which is why they help hold your hair in place. Unfortunately, they also hold dirt and oil in place, which dulls your hair's clean appearance.

Hair spray. Of course, there's always good old hair spray. Actually, hair sprays have improved greatly in recent years. No longer do they shellac your hair together, unless you use stronger-holding, stiffening sprays. There's also good news if you want to do your part in preventing further damage to the ozone layer: Most hair spray is available in nonaerosol containers.

Regardless of what you put on your hair to hold it in place, remember, you are putting something sticky on your clean hair. If you allow that sticky product to build up, your hair will soon feel like a mattress. To avoid this mess, every few weeks or so, I mix a bit of baking soda in with my shampoo. This cuts through the product buildup and gives my hair a great, clean look and feel.

Try to let your hair go natural whenever possible. Sometimes I'll just wash and dry my hair without putting any other products on it. The "breather" really seems to help.

PERMS

I've always felt that perms, or permanents, were misnamed. If a perm is permanent, why do we have to get them so often? Okay, I won't be so technical since a perm does put extra body, fullness, or curl into your hair for a much longer period of time than any other artificial means.

Perms, partial perms, and body waves all work basically the same way. A chemical lotion is applied to your hair while it is in rollers and allowed to "set." The amount of time required varies according to the product.

Then, with your hair still in rollers, a neutralizer is applied. This causes your hair to take on the new curled or waved position which it will retain until it grows out or is relaxed.

Permanents can be done by your hairdresser, which is usually safer and more effective, but also more expensive. Or, you can have a perm done at home. Home permanent horror stories abound, but mostly the mistakes are because of "human error" rather than product malfunctions. If you and the person helping you follow the instructions carefully, home permanents can be fun and effective.

Here are a few things to remember about permed hair:

1. Don't shampoo for at least forty-eight hours after you have permed your hair.

2. Processing your hair (perming, waving, coloring, or straightening) can dry your hair. You will need special shampoos and conditioners that are designed for processed hair. Processed hair is often very fragile; it needs regular conditioning to make up for the moisture it loses in the processing.

3. If you blow-dry your perm, keep the dryer on a low heat setting.

4. Use a wide-toothed comb when combing wet, permed hair, in order to avoid split ends or other breakage.

What are some ways you've discovered that help you "stay" where you need to be with the Lord?

Life is ten percent what you make it and ninety percent how you take it.

IRVING BERLIN

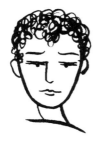

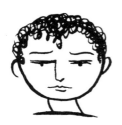

THE RIGHT CUT FOR YOU

The good news is that cleansing, conditioning, and contouring your hair can make a good haircut look terrific. The bad news is that all of my "C-crets" to great-looking hair will be wasted if your haircut looks as though your great Aunt Matilda put a bowl on your head and just trimmed around the edges. A couple of factors should be considered before you get your next haircut: your body size, your face shape, and your life-style.

There are no set rules when it comes to matching your haircut with your height and weight. Your best bet is probably to experiment and find the style most flattering and comfortable for you. There are a few things to keep in mind, however. Many fashion models, for example, are quite tall and have short, closely cropped hair. On the other hand, a girl I know, Dorrene, is short and rather pudgy, yet she, too, wears her hair short and closely cropped. On Dorrene, the shorter haircut tends to draw attention to her pudginess; a slightly longer, fuller style might soften and balance her overall appearance.

The shape of your face also influences to a large degree what hairstyle will look best on you. My face almost demands that I wear a short style. Even when my hair was at its longest, I still pulled it back, off my ears, to fit better with my face shape.

Obviously, no two faces are identical (not even with identical twins), but your face is probably similar to one of the seven basic shapes: square, rectangle, pear, round, oval, heart, and oblong or diamond. For better or worse, many makeup and hairstyling techniques attempt to give you an oval shape. The best thing to remember when choosing a hairstyle is that you don't want it to repeat the shape of your face.

For example, if you have a round face, you'd be wise to avoid a short, curly hairstyle. It will only exaggerate the roundness of your face. A longer, straighter hairstyle would move you more toward an oval look. If your face is square or rectangular, you'll want to avoid a cut that emphasizes your jaw and forehead. If your face is oblong, you may want to add fullness to the cheekbone area and avoid a longer, straight cut.

Again, there are no set rules, especially nowadays, when it comes to hairstyles, but try to choose a cut that compliments your height, weight, and face.

Your life-style should also be considered before deciding on your haircut. Are you active in sports? Perhaps a shorter, easier-to-care-for style may be preferable to lengthy locks. Try to find a style that matches your time limits and one that can be changed with minimal effort in order to fit your various activities, whether "dressing up" or "dressing down."

How to Pick a Hairstylist

If your goal is to get as good a haircut as possible, I strongly advise going to a styling professional. Don't even think about trying to cut your own hair! Usually, letting a friend take the shears to your hair is a mistake, too, unless your friend is a professional stylist.

Yes, good stylists cost money, and the better ones are usually even more expensive. If you want to save money on your haircut, go to the best stylist you can afford, but have him or her cut your hair a little shorter than necessary. Or try to stretch the time between haircuts. If your hair is short, instead of getting your hair trimmed once every three or four weeks, go for a full cut once every six to eight weeks. With longer styles, you can

The Lord is the "Master Stylist." What things do you feel He wants to "cut out of your life?" What areas does He seem to want to shape?

allow even more time between cuts. Just don't scrimp on your hairstylist.

And whatever you do, don't walk into a styling salon and say, "Here I am. Do whatever you think looks good." You may come out with a lot less hair than you thought. At least give some thought to how you would like to look before you go stylist shopping.

Similarly, don't just pick a stylist's name out of the phone book or from an advertisement. Ask around a little. Personal recommendations are still the best way to find a stylist. Look for someone who has helped a friend of yours find the right "look." Of course, if your friend's stylist's customers all look similar, you may want to keep looking . . . unless you really like your friend's look.

The first time you visit the stylist's shop, be sure to wear your hair the way you normally do. In some salons, a person other than the stylist may be given the responsibility of washing your hair before you get it cut. If so, ask to see the stylist who will cut your hair ahead of time, before your hair is sopping wet, so he or she can get a picture of your current cut.

Remember, your stylist is not a mind reader. He or she doesn't know your hair-care preferences or past problems. You need to let your stylist know what sort of look you hope to achieve and what type of life-style you lead. For example, if you have to be at school or work every morning at eight o'clock, you may not want a hairstyle that is going to cost you an hour of preparation time each day. If your stylist is unwilling to consider such personal details, find yourself another stylist. A good stylist knows that a great haircut is useless if it doesn't work with your life-style.

Also, avoid being a passive spectator in your stylist's chair. While you must give the stylist an opportunity to work, don't be bashful about expressing your opinions concerning the cut. If you want more or less cut off, say so. There's not much use complaining after the fact. "Wow! I didn't really want it that short!" Remember, it's your hair; you're the one who is going to have to live with it, not your stylist.

As for what style best suits you, I'd say go with the flow. In other words, whether you have curly hair, a "widow's peak," straight hair, or hair with a complete mind of its own, go with the natural direction your hair is flowing. This is especially important if you don't have the time or desire for a lot of hair upkeep. Instead of fighting against what God gave you on top of your head, you'll save a lot of time, money, and energy if you work with your natural characteristics rather than in opposition to them.

Idolatry is worshiping anything that ought to be used, or using anything that is meant to be worshiped.
AUGUSTINE

COLOR MY WORLD

Although I don't recommend that young girls color their hair, by the time they are in high school, many young women want to add some color, add highlights, or lighten their hair. Be careful here. Your first question should be, "Why?" Why do you want to alter your hair color?

Many young women believe that by changing their hair color, they can change their personalities. It doesn't happen that way. Like I said at the beginning of this book, whatever is going on inside of you has a way of showing up in your appearance. No number of exterior paint jobs will make you feel better about yourself. You've got to start working from the inside, out.

"But I'm bored with the way I look!" many young women respond in answer to the "why" question. "I just want to try something different." Trust me. I know the feeling. I've tried just about every "natural" hair color possible, but I always come back to one that is close to my natural color.

There's nothing wrong with experimenting. Just remember, though, the Master Stylist created your hair color to match your eyes, skin tone, and skin type, and He's been doing a huge business for ages. If you are hoping to turn into somebody else by coloring your hair, forget it. God made you to be you.

Experimenting with new looks can be fun; just don't overdo it. Changing your hair color can also add some shine and body to your hair. If at some point you do consider coloring your hair, here are a few tips you need to know.

First, you'll get the best results if you keep your new hair color close to your natural color. Second, I strongly suggest getting professional help. Very few women are adept enough to color, highlight, or process their own hair.

If you can't afford to have a professional color your hair, but you still want to "do something" to your hair color, the first and foremost rule is READ THE LABELS ON THE PACKAGE! This is especially important, because various hair-coloring products are meant to last longer than others. Whatever type of coloring you decide to use, follow the directions to the letter.

Everybody wants to be normal but nobody wants to be average.
MARY MCDONALD

TEMPORARY COLORS

Temporary colors are the gentlest on your hair and can be tons of fun if you just want to experiment with a new color. This type of coloring will wash out with your next shampoo. You can purchase these products in a rinse, mousse, or a shampoo. If you are tentatively testing the possibilities of hair coloring, temporary colors are for you. Understand, though, these products are not designed to take you all the way from dark brunette to blonde. Their effects are much more subtle.

One caution concerning temporary tints. Don't put one in your hair the night before you have physical education class or before you plan to go swimming. Remember, these colors really do come out in the wash!

SEMIPERMANENT COLORS

The name says it all. These colors usually last anywhere from four to six shampoos. Each time you shampoo, a little more color will come out. The good news is that it comes out relatively evenly. This is because some of the semipermanent color seeps through your hair's cuticle and into the cortex. This will not harm your hair, but as you wash it, the colors wash out of the cortex, and before long, you will have to reapply the color if you want to keep it. Again, these colors will disappoint you if you are looking for a radical change.

PERMANENT COLORS

This is the product you want if you are looking for long-term, extreme change to your hair. But be forewarned: they don't call these dyes and bleaches permanent without reason. These colors will remain until you cut off the colored hair or strip the color off with chemicals designed for that purpose. Meanwhile, your roots will be pushing your original hair color back into sight. Also, before using any dyes or tints, you should give yourself a "patch" test. Hair dyes contain strong chemicals which could cause swelling, itching, and general discomfort

Nothing is a greater impediment to being on good terms with others than being ill at ease with yourself.

HONORÉ DE BALZAC

around your face. The medical term for this is contact dermatitis. Also, be aware that double processing (perming and coloring) your hair requires special treatment. Again, seek help from a professional before attempting to color permed hair or to perm colored hair.

To make sure you won't be adversely affected by coloring your hair, mix a capful of peroxide with a capful of the coloring you wish to use. Wash and dry an area of skin behind your ear; then, using a cotton swab or a Q-tip, apply the mixture to about a one-inch square of your skin. Now wait one full day.

If your skin shows any negative reaction within the twenty-four hours—itching, redness, soreness, anything—do not use the product. You may be able to use other coloring products (try a product by a different company), but that one will do much more than color your hair if you go ahead and use it!

Obviously, you want to thoroughly think through this move before you put permanent coloring in your hair. I didn't one time, and wow! Did I ever feel silly.

One day my friend and fashion adviser, Joan Tankersley, and I went into a wig shop in Hollywood. It was the day before we were to shoot the photographs for my second album cover, and we were just goofing off and having fun. On a whim, I tried on a beautiful, curly, red wig. The response was overwhelming. People in the shop started oooing and ahhing, telling me how gorgeous the red wig looked.

We had just come from one of Hollywood's finer hair salons where I'd had my hair highlighted for the album pictures. Nevertheless, Joan was ecstatic.

"Come on, Kim!" she coaxed. "Let's go back right now and tell them you want your hair to be red."

"Joan, I can't do that! I can't make that sort of

decision today and turn up with red hair tomorrow for an album shoot."

Joan kept insisting, but I kept refusing. For the next year, she refused to relent. She kept reminding me, "Kim, remember how great you looked with that red hair?" By the time we were ready to take the photos for my next album cover, she had talked me into it.

We went to one of the top hair salons in Los Angeles. When Joan and I told them what we wanted them to do, the stylists all gushed, "Oh, yes! Red hair would be gorgeous on you."

I sat in their salon for six hours while they transformed my hair color to red. Since my hair was highlighted, the stylists first had to put color back into my hair. To do so, they put in a gaudy, awful-looking color of red, somewhere between Ronald McDonald, Lucille Ball, and Raggedy Ann. It was horrible!

"Wait a minute! Wait a minute," the stylists consoled me when they saw the shocked expression on my face as I looked in the mirror. "That's just the filler," they explained, attempting to calm my fears. They then went to work at putting a beautiful, auburn-burgundy color in my hair, and when they were finally done, I had to admit, it looked fabulous. But it just wasn't me.

For weeks, every time I'd walk by a mirror, I'd do a double take, wondering, Who is that woman? It was beautiful hair, but I never really got used to it. Neither did my family.

Besides that, it was terribly difficult to keep up. My hair would look great for about three weeks, but since it was blonde underneath, it would start to fade and look really awful for three months. When it came time for the next album photo shoot, I said, "I can't take this red thing anymore," and had my hair rinsed back to a color

Have you ever allowed a friend's opinion to influence you to the point of doing something that you didn't really like?
What would be a better way to handle that sort of situation?

closer to my natural hair color.

Experimenting with your hair can be fun, but always go with what works for you (even if your best friend says, "You'd look incredible with purple hair!"). Because in order to look your best, you've got to feel good about yourself.

THAT DIRTY "D" WORD

WHAT CAUSES DANDRUFF?

God is our refuge and strength, an ever-present help in trouble.

Therefore we will not fear, though the earth give way and the mountains fall into the heart of the sea.

PSALM 46:1,2 (NIV)

Dermatologists don't know a great deal about dandruff, and I doubt whether they truly care to. After all, ridding the world of dandruff doesn't exactly rank up there with finding a cure for cancer, heart disease, or AIDS. Still, when you've suffered through enough lonely evenings, itching and scratching your scalp, or brushing flakes off your shoulders, you're about ready to will your body to science so somebody can discover a solution!

Some dandruff really is caused by skin diseases. Psoriasis, seborrhea, and other scalp diseases require medical attention, not merely a new shampoo.

Sometimes dandruff can be related to tension and stress in your life. Tension usually causes your sebaceous glands (remember them?) to work overtime, producing an excess of oil on your skin and scalp. That's why before a big test or before a long-awaited date, your face often breaks out and your shoulders look as though you just came inside out of a snowstorm.

A "psuedo-dandruff" can also result from using too much hair spray or other styling products. Although the hair products themselves do not cause dandruff, if you use too much, the product flakes off when you comb or brush your hair and makes it look as though you have the real thing.

Most dandruff, however, seems to be caused by one of two culprits: a scalp that is too oily, or a scalp that is too dry. Either one, you'll be glad to know, is easily corrected.

OILY-SCALP DANDRUFF

Somebody ought to write a song, "Blame It on Your Sebaceous Glands!" Well, maybe not. But when those overactive "S" glands of yours produce too much oil, your scalp cells get irritated, which then, in self-defense, speed up their growth (and death) cycle. The dried, dead cells get stuck in the excess oil then clump together and flake off as dandruff.

To rid yourself of this sort of dandruff, you must remove the dead cells and the oil. *Great*, you're probably thinking. *How do I do that?*

A good, over-the-counter dandruff shampoo that contains sulfur should do the job. Use the dandruff shampoo only until you get your dandruff under control. Contrary to certain television commercials touting dandruff shampoos for regular use, prolonged use of these shampoos (if they are truly effective) can actually make your scalp worse.

Once your dandruff has been eliminated, all you need to do is use a shampoo formulated for oily hair. Keep your hair clean and well-brushed, and you should have little trouble with dandruff. If you do spot signs of trouble, go back to the dandruff shampoo again for a while.

For extra protection, try conditioning your hair with a lemon rinse. Squeeze the juice from one lemon into a cup of lukewarm water. Then after you shampoo, pour the lemon and water onto your hair, just as you would any other conditioner. Work it through your hair and scalp. Then rinse it out with cool water. This closes the pores on

Life is either a daring adventure or nothing.
HELEN KELLER

your scalp, causing less oil to slip out. The lemon rinse does wonders for oily hair whether you have dandruff or not. Try it!

DRY-SCALP DANDRUFF

If your scalp lacks moisture, dandruff may be the result. To put it simply, if your scalp is dry, the cells on the surface have nothing they can hang onto; consequently, they fall off as flakes of dandruff.

To correct this problem, first you must get rid of the flakes, then you must moisturize your scalp. Getting rid of the flakes is the easy part. Many of the popular dandruff shampoos will do this for you. Getting the moisture into your scalp takes a little more effort.

Try this: Warm three or four tablespoons of some hand or body lotion, being careful not to get it too hot. Then work it into your hair, all the way down to your scalp. Run hot water over a towel, wring it out, and while it is still warm, wrap it around your head. Keep it on for about twenty minutes. Then wash your hair with a mild dandruff shampoo or a shampoo made especially for dry hair.

He who ignores discipline despises himself, but whoever heeds correction gains understanding.
PROVERBS 15:32 (NIV)

LAZY-BONES DANDRUFF

Although this is not a medically accurate term, "lazy-bones dandruff" can occur if you slack off in your hair care. By not brushing your hair, not shampooing well enough, or not rinsing thoroughly, you are simply inviting those dead cells to hang out together until they get blown off your head. In order to keep your scalp clean and healthy, you must maintain proper hair care.

PROCESSED HAIR: A PARTICULAR DANDRUFF PROBLEM

If you have permed, straightened, colored, or otherwise "processed" hair, dandruff can be a particularly sticky problem for you. Many effective dandruff shampoos use sulfur or other strong medications to eliminate the dandruff. Unfortunately, sulfur frequently causes processed hair to tangle, mat, and even clump together in a sticky mess of mangled hair.

Often this lump of hair can be removed only by cutting it out, which can leave an unsightly swath three or four inches wide in your hair. User beware! If you have processed hair and you notice some dandruff, use an extremely mild dandruff shampoo. Again, READ THE LABELS CAREFULLY! Make sure that the shampoo you select is safe to use on processed hair, unless of course, you happen to like the Mohawk look.

Look for dandruff shampoos that contain zinc rather than sulfur. Head and Shoulders (Procter & Gamble) is an example of a dandruff shampoo that uses zinc pyrithione rather than sulfur.

Although dandruff doesn't hurt, it can be a real pain. Nevertheless, most dandruff is controllable. It may take a little time and effort to keep your scalp clean and smooth, but believe me, it's well worth it.

She was an intelligent and beautifull woman. . . .
(DESCRIPTION OF ABAGAIL, I SAMUEL 25:3 NIV)

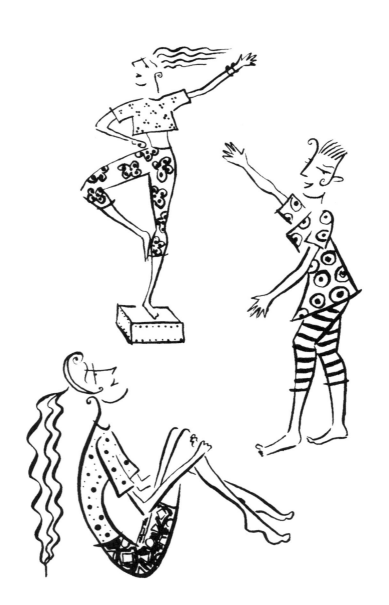

No Body Is Perfect

THERE ARE LOTS OF THINGS I LOVE TO DO, but dieting is not one of them. I've never been a successful dieter. At one point in my life, I was seventeen pounds heavier than I am now. Dieting didn't work for me, but a change of life-style did.

I didn't do anything major. I just began thinking, *I've got to do something about this. What can I change? How can I eat healthier?* I began making small, barely perceptible changes in my eating habits, but those slight changes gradually brought about major long-term benefits.

For me, an obvious place to begin was dessert. I love desserts! Who doesn't? But I decided, *Okay, if I am going to have a dessert, what is my least-fattening option?*

Instead of eating ice cream, for example, I now eat frozen yogurt. It has nearly as many calories as ice cream, but nowhere near the amount of sugar and fat. If I am at a restaurant, instead of ordering that huge piece of chocolate cake, covered with icing and syrup, I'll ask for strawberries with a light whipped cream. See, no big deal. I'm just making minor adjustments in my eating habits, and they are paying great dividends.

Do I ever blow it? You bet I do! Big-time! Sometimes I'll go for the chocolate cake and the ice cream. But I've discovered a few patterns, and recognizing my weaknesses has helped me to avoid over-eating. For instance, I've noticed that if I'm eating alone, I tend to eat more. Also, if I'm eating out of boredom, I sometimes will eat things that I know are not the best for me. If I have cooked the meal, I might overdo it. After all, I went to all the trouble to cook that food . . .

When I blow my normal eating habits, I don't punish myself or starve myself in an attempt to make up for my mistake. On the other hand, I do make every effort to get back on track the next day.

Steve Silva, fitness director of Health Management Resources in Boston, says losing weight or maintaining your current weight doesn't have to be difficult at all; it's just a matter of lowering the fat in your diet.[1] For example, by simply substituting three glasses of skim (or low-fat) milk for three glasses of whole milk every day, in one year you could lose about fifteen pounds!

Furthermore, by eating two pieces of whole-wheat

There are no ordinary people.
C. S. LEWIS
THE WEIGHT OF GLORY

toast rather than a doughnut every morning, you could lose twelve pounds in twelve months. Those little things make a big difference!

WHO SAYS SLIM IS IN?

Unfortunately, most of our society. God created your body, and He thinks you are pretty incredible just the way you are! He loves you, accepts you, and values you immensely, whether you are a size four or a size fourteen. Your worth as an individual has absolutely nothing to do with the size or shape of your body. The most important thing about you is not how you look, but who you are. It is important to take care of your body and maintain a healthy weight, but the super slim look that the media pushes as beautiful is not always healthy.

I never laugh at fat people. One shouldn't laugh at other's expanse.
SHELBY FRIEDMAN

Everywhere you look in our society, we are bombarded with the message that a slim, svelte body is attractive. Despite television stars such as Oprah Winfrey, Roseanne (Barr) Arnold, Delta Burke, and others who say that they are "free to be fat," or those who herald that "heftiness is happiness," you and I both know that in your school or office, it probably isn't that way.

Slim wasn't always in, though. Years ago, it was just the opposite. Browse through any art gallery, and you might be surprised at the number of plump women depicted in famous paintings. In many Middle Eastern countries yet today, the belly dancers considered most attractive are chunky by western standards. Even in Hawaii, island home of the hula, the genuine hula girls appear grossly overweight when compared to the slick, sleek images displayed on TV or in tourist traps.

Sure, I believe we ought to try our best to look good, but not so we can compare with or conform to

Nothing is important but that which is eternal.

Amy Carmichael

Kohila

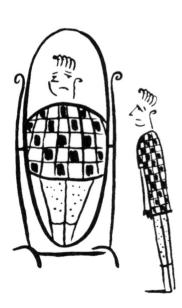

our society's warped ideas of beauty. We have a responsibility to take care of our bodies because we represent our King Jesus. Moreover, it is our relationship with Him that ultimately gives us a sense of who we are—children of God! We are His unique creations, each one a never-to-be-repeated masterpiece!

My husband, Gary, and I attend a Bible study at our church every Tuesday morning when we are at home in Nashville. One day the discussion turned to the balance between being pretty (or handsome) and being proud. Our pastor, L. H. Hardwick, put the subject into perspective for me. He said, "God doesn't mind you being as pretty as you can be, but He doesn't want you to desire to be prettier than somebody else."

Most teenage young women I meet nowadays think they are overweight. Many of them are not. They have been led into believing that they must measure up to somebody else's standards, that they should look like the women they see in the movies, on television, or in the fashion magazines. Some girls who see themselves as fat and unattractive start taking laxatives, diet pills, or water pills to help them lose weight. They risk becoming victims of anorexia nervosa or bulimia, eating disorders that are common among people obsessed with losing weight.

Anorexia victims lose their desire to eat. Even though their weight may be normal or below normal, they view themselves as being fat and grossly overweight, so they stop eating. On the other hand, bulimia victims often eat in binges, gorging themselves with food, and then self-induce vomiting.

Both of these eating disorders are serious and can lead to other ailments, even death. The causes of anorexia and bulimia are often complex and numerous.

Many who suffer from eating disorders have a desperate need to feel loved. They need to know that God's love for them and His acceptance of them is not contingent upon their looks or their weight!

If you find yourself obsessed with food or think you might have an eating disorder, please talk to someone. It is not an easy thing to do, but there are lots of people who are able, willing, and want to help. If you're not sure where to start, your youth pastor or pastor can listen, and your guidance counselor at school probably has lots of information and would be able to help. And most of all, don't forget that God is always available and always listening.

For God so loved the world, that he gave his only begotten Son, that whosoever believeth in him should not perish, but have everlasting life.

JOHN 3:16 (KJV)

WHAT CAUSES A WEIGHT PROBLEM?

If you really are overweight (or underweight) as determined by a medical doctor, a number of factors may contribute to your diet problems. Here are a few of the more common ones:

1. *Television.* No, the TV itself can't cause you to be overweight (unless you run out, buy, and eat all the fattening foods that are advertised on the tube— deep-fried foods, beef products, soda pop, ice cream, corn chips, and lots of others). But if you are a TV-aholic, you are probably eating a bunch of junk food, as well. Furthermore, you most likely are lacking in exercise. A couch potato burns extremely few calories flicking the remote control.

   The average teenager watches twenty-five hours of TV each week. If you reduce that amount by only two hours, and substitute a half hour to forty-five minutes of exercise three times each week, you might be amazed at the results.

2. *Fast-Food Favorites.* It is no secret that most fast-food

My body retains ice cream.
ZIG ZIGLAR
KEYNOTE SPEECH, *1989*
NATIONAL SPEAKERS ASSOC.
CONVENTION

restaurants target teenagers. And actually, the love affair is mutual. Most guys and girls love burgers, pizza, pop, French fries, ice cream, tacos, fried chicken, and roast beef sandwiches. Unfortunately, most fast foods are loaded with calories, not to mention fat and salt.

I'm not knocking fast-food restaurants; in fact, I'm grateful for them! When Gary and I are on the road with our band, because of our hectic schedule we are frequently forced to stop at a fast-food place and grab a quick bite to eat.

Usually, I head straight for the salad bar. I load up on lettuce, vegetables, fruit, and use only a small amount of dressing. Even the low-cal stuff is chock full of calories. They ought to call it "lower-cal." I skip right past the potato salads—they're usually full of highly fattening mayonnaise.

If I do have a sandwich, I ask for the simplest they have; I rarely order a deluxe burger or sandwich. I try to avoid French fries, onion rings, or anything else that is deep-fried. I also skip most pastas and tartar sauces.

Fortunately, many fast-food chains are now offering some sort of lean menu. While some of the entreés are rather bland, many of the leaner items are quite tasty. Most fast-food chains now offer skinless, grilled chicken, too. If it is not fried or coated in mayonnaise, a chicken sandwich is lower in calories than most burgers.

Given a choice, Gary and I go for pizza over a burger anytime. A piece of pizza is pretty healthy and is lower in fat than a burger-and-fries combo. Of course, if you eat the entire pizza "pie," the calories can add up quickly.

3. *Emotional Stress.* Another factor that causes many people to overeat is stress. Stress can strike you from any number of sources: your parents pressuring you about your grades or to get a summer job, your friends, your teachers, sports or academic competition, or your social life!

It's not what you eat, it's what's eating you.
(BOOK TITLE)

Some individuals attempt to deal with stress by smoking, drinking, or doing drugs. These dangerous crutches only exacerbate the problem. Many young women turn to food in times of trouble. As the old saying puts it, "When the going gets tough, the tough go out for ice cream" . . . or something like that.

Quoted in an article in *Harper's Bazaar*, Dr. Ellen McGrath, director of the Psychology Center in New York City and Newport Beach, Calif., concurs, "I would estimate that some 80 percent of the women I've seen [as patients] use food to get them through a tough time." [2]

If you find that you tend to overeat in times of stress, try to talk with your parents about it. Perhaps it would help to have a good, heart-to-heart talk with a close friend, or your church youth leader or pastor. Don't be ashamed to ask for help. We all get stressed out from time to time. It helps to talk about it.

Remember, the best friend you'll ever have is Jesus. Even if you feel you can't talk to anyone else, you can talk to Him. He is always available to you, and He would love to talk with you. Go ahead; pour out your heart to Him, and be sure to listen when He speaks to you, as well.

4. *Your Body Type.* Although this is not actually a cause of weight problems, an obvious but often overlooked factor in weight discussions is your basic body type.

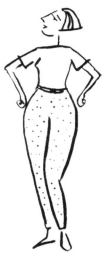

PEAR-SHAPED

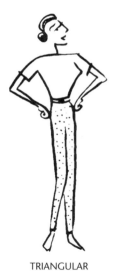

TRIANGULAR

Without getting too technical, most women are born with one of four body shapes: pear, triangular, box, or hourglass. The shapes are pretty self-explanatory and are so described depending upon how a woman's body stores and distributes fat.

The *pear-shaped* body normally has narrow shoulders, a small bust line, and wide hips. Fat tends to be stored around the hips and thighs, often leading to the unflattering nickname, "thunderthighs."

A person with a *triangular* body shape has wide shoulders that taper to a tiny waist. Fat collects in the upper body, causing a sort of barrel-chested look.

A woman with a *box* body shape has a rather straight-line structure. Her hips and bust line are flatter, and the fat is distributed more evenly throughout her body.

The *hourglass figure* is not merely a figment of Hollywood's imagination. A woman with this body shape has a smaller waist, and her hip and bust measurements are nearly the same. Fat drifts toward her upper body and lower body, but not to her waist or midriff.

The Lord gave you one of these shapes, and, apart from major cosmetic surgery (which I do not recommend!), there's not a lot you can change about it. But by eating healthy and exercising, you can make the most of what you have.

Everyone has a unique bone structure. We all carry weight differently. That is why it is extremely foolish to compare your weight with the weight of anyone else.

My friend and former band member Dana Glover is a fashion model for a top New York agency.

She weighs twenty pounds more than I do, but then she's a full six inches taller than I am! Dana looks fabulous, but for me to attempt to match her pound for pound would be ridiculous.

5. *Thank You, Mom and Dad.* As with most of your physical characteristics, heredity plays a major part. If your parents are overweight, guess what? Yep. There is a high probability that you will follow in their footsteps. Part of this, of course, can be explained by genetics and is out of your control. On the other hand, your pudgies may have more to do with the fact that Mom is a great cook, or that your family members continue to stock the refrigerator and cupboards with fattening foods. That part is controllable, though admittedly, not easy.

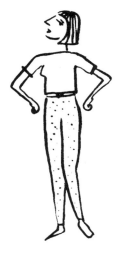

BOX

If your parents and other family members are junk food junkies or have horrible eating habits, it will probably be harder for you to adjust your own food intake, but it's not impossible. Perhaps you can make some low-fat meal suggestions, or better yet, offer to make the meal yourself. You could also suggest that the family switch to low-fat milk. Hey, every little calorie-saving idea helps!

Why not ask your family members to fill their plates at the stove and carry them to the dining area? People are less prone to take seconds (you included) when they have to go back to the serving area to get it.

You could also offer to do the family's grocery shopping. That way, you can purchase foods that are lower in calories and snacks that are healthier and less fattening. Yes! They do exist—try some popcorn, frozen yogurt, vanilla wafers, or oatmeal cookies.

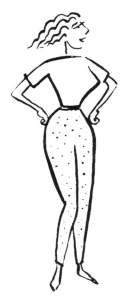

HOURGLASS FIGURE

Dieters try to dispose of their hazardous waists.

DIETS, DIETS EVERYWHERE!

If you do decide to "go on a diet," be sure to check with your doctor first. Have him or her design a diet that is safe and appropriate for you. A safe program should cause you to lose no more than one or two pounds per week.

Whatever you do, avoid fad diets. Nowadays, it seems a new diet craze hits the television talk show circuit as soon as the last one disappears. In the past few years, people have extolled the virtues of the Scarsdale Diet, the Stillman Diet, the water diet, the "eat-all-the-ice-cream-you-can-stuff-in-your-body diet" (I made that one up!), the Rotation Diet, the T-Factor Diet, the magic powder diets, and countless others. Support groups, diet clubs, and expensive weight-loss programs have proliferated. Although most of these programs have some merit, all fad diets are doomed to failure. Yes, you may lose weight for a while, but "statistics show that a whopping ninety percent of the people who lose pounds from fad diets, gain the weight back within a year."[3]

How can you tell if a food program is a fad diet or a rip-off? It's probably a bad diet if:

- It promises "effortless" results, with no change in your eating habits or life-style.
- It guarantees fast weight-loss.
- It requires pills, vitamins, or other drugs to speed up your metabolism.
- It doesn't include foods from the four major food groups: meats, milk products, fruits and vegetables, and breads and cereals.
- It's called a "miracle diet" or hailed as a "new discovery" in weight-loss programs.

The truth is that in order to lose weight and keep it

off, you must transform your life-style in two vital areas:

1. You must establish healthy eating habits.
2. You must establish a reasonable, workable, regular exercise regimen.

FOOD FOR FITNESS

Let's talk about food first. I'm not a dietician, so I won't even try to prescribe a proper diet for you. Nevertheless, of one thing I am certain: if you hope to get control of a runaway weight problem, you must establish healthy eating habits. For starters, plan on eating three meals a day. Most teens don't. They blow off breakfast, scarf down a fast lunch, then pig out on dinner, snacks, or junk food later in the day. If they were to eat three balanced meals each day, they'd be much better off.

"What?" I can almost hear you protesting. "I want to control my weight, not begin looking like the Goodyear Blimp!"

Never fear. Many people are unsuccessful at dieting because they are hungry all the time. Profound, huh? But it's true. In order for your diet plan to work, you must feel full and not feel that you are depriving yourself of your favorite foods. A proper food program will do that for you; it will include breakfast, lunch, and dinner, and will even recommend nonfattening desserts. That way you won't be hungry. If you are constantly enduring hunger pangs while on a diet, that diet is wrong for you.

Don't skip meals in your attempt to lose weight. When you skip meals or snacks, it becomes increasingly difficult to conquer your hunger as the day goes on. Frequently, dieters who skip meals during the daylight hours will cheat after dark. Most dieticians say that ideally, you should have consumed two thirds of your total daily calorie intake before sundown.

The trick to this three-meal-per-day plan is to eat

My loss of weight was due to exercise, hard work, and diet, which proves that people will go to great lengths to avoid great widths.

ERNEST BORGNINE

The rot is in all of us, for how many of us would be willing to divide our riches among our own family, let alone the poor or needy, beyond, of course, what we can easily afford—for if we were willing, why have we not done it?

COLIN TURNBULL,
ANTHROPOLOGIST
THE MOUNTAIN PEOPLE

Never eat more than you can lift.
MISS PIGGY

only the foods your dietician prescribes for you, and you must eat properly sized portions. Lora, a sophomore in high school, is trying to lose about twenty pounds, but has not been having much success.

"I don't understand it," she laments. "All I have for lunch every day is a salad and a diet drink, but I'm not making any progress."

Lora's problem is that she loads up her plate with a mountain of lettuce, then covers it with cheese, ham, croutons, raisins, and other high-calorie goodies. Then she coats the entire thing with a thick layer of rich salad dressing. (One tablespoon of regular salad dressing can be 75 to 100 calories!) By the time Lora is finished, her "dietetic" salad is pushing the 1000 calorie mark. On a 1200 to 1500 calorie per day diet, she has already eaten two thirds of her allowable intake. By supper time, she feels as though she is starving and plunges right into the meal along with the rest of her family, postponing her diet for another day.

WHAT CAN I EAT?

While I can't give you a precise plan, I can tell you that certain foods are better for you than others, if you are trying to stick to a low-fat diet. Foods such as chicken and fish are more healthy than beef products. Fruits are great. Vegetables are also great, but don't give your veggies a butter bath or coat them in fattening sauces. Three or four eggs each week are okay; three or four eggs per day . . . that's a different story.

Melon produce is good for you, and so are vegetable or fruit juices as long as they are not saturated with sugar. Potatoes are extremely nutritious, and they aren't fattening . . . until you start packing your baked potato with butter, sour cream, broccoli and cheese, or other diet busters.

Black coffee and tea are okay, as far as calories go, but they do stain your teeth, and the jury is still out on what java's caffeine does to your heart. Low-fat or skim milk is better for you; whole milk will pour on the pounds.

WHAT FOODS TO AVOID

Foods high in sugar and fat are bad for your diet. If you are serious about losing weight or maintaining your present weight, you will want to avoid red meat, foods with lots of refined (white) sugar, lots of dairy products (you need the calcium and other nutrients found in milk, so go for the skim rather than two-percent or whole milk), any foods that are deep-fried or have palm oil, and of course, everybody's favorite—junk food. (Ever wonder why they call it junk?) I'm not saying you should never have any of these foods—everyone needs a treat once in a while—but if they are a regular part of your diet, you are going to have a tough time losing weight.

Is not life more than food?
MATTHEW 6:25

Again, alcoholic beverages are a no-no. While they are bad for you in other ways, beer, wine, and mixed drinks add tons of calories to your diet. Personally, I am an abstainer, for both spiritual and health reasons.

Other items to avoid include sweetened soft drinks (diet drinks aren't great for you either—they are high in sodium and caffeine), butter, hot cakes, sweet rolls, sugar-coated cereals, most cheese products except for cottage cheese (that slice of cheese you put on your sandwich can add a quick 100 calories!), puddings, creamy sauces, or soups.

You may be thinking, "You're telling me to avoid all

my favorites!" I know. I know. I didn't say it would be easy. The average teenager needs between 2000 and 2500 calories a day. If you want to lose one pound per week, you will probably need to knock off about 500 calories every day. If you want to gain one pound each week, you will need to add 500 calories per day to your diet. I am not a compulsive calorie counter, and I am not encouraging you to become one either, but just making a conscious effort to control what we eat will help.

I don't worry much about weighing myself, either. I may step onto the scale once a month or so, but as long as I feel good about myself and like what I see when I look in the mirror, I don't pay much attention to the number on the scale.

DO I REALLY HAVE TO EXERCISE?

Yep. The second essential ingredient to any weight-loss program is exercise. Cutting calories without combining that effort with an exercise program does not normally lead to permanent weight loss. In fact, current research shows just the opposite, that trying to lose weight without establishing a consistent exercise regimen is next to impossible. A study done by Scott Weigle, M.D., at the University of Washington in Seattle, discovered that, "Overweight adults on a low-calorie diet found that their bodies adjusted to the reduced food intake by the end of the diet."[4] Without exercise, the participants put the weight back on in hardly no time at all.

There are a few reasons that happens. First, as you reduce the number of calories you consume, your body's metabolism slows down so it burns fewer calories, actually making it harder for you to lose weight.

Second, the pounds that you do lose by simply cutting calories are often made up of crucial muscle

The only exercise some people get is jumping to conclusions, running down their friends, sidestepping responsibility, dodging issues, passing the buck, and pushing their luck.
BAPTIST COURIER

mass, not just fat. Your muscles burn calories, so the less muscle you have, the fewer calories you will burn in the long run, and the less weight you will lose.

Third, even though you may lose weight for a while by simply cutting calories, your body still "thinks" that it needs the same number of calories as before. As such, as soon as you begin to eat normally, even if you eat healthy foods and avoid the fattening stuff, your body begins to store fat, and you will begin to gain weight.

This cycle of weight loss and gain, sometimes called "the yo-yo effect," is hard on your heart, your blood pressure, and your blood-sugar levels, not to mention what it does to your self-image. Short-term complications from low-calorie diets without exercise may include constipation, fatigue, dizziness, muscle cramping, and headaches.

That's why the combination of cutting calories and working out is a more effective way to bring about permanent weight loss. As I said before, a change in life-style is what we are talking about, not simply the shedding of a few pounds.

Working out helps your body burn calories faster. It also helps your body improve or maintain its muscle tone, which burns more calories, making weight loss that much quicker.

A balanced program of proper diet and exercise actually makes the entire process of weight loss easier. If you think about this, it just makes sense. Say you need to drop 500 calories a day in order to lose a pound per week. If you burn 250 calories per day by exercising, you are halfway there, and you haven't changed a thing about your diet yet. Now knock out 250 calories per day of those fattening foods and you are on your way to a trimmer, healthier body.

Exercise is an important part of our lives, but it should not be the most important part. Maybe that's why Paul wrote to the young man, Timothy: "Spend your time and energy in the exercise of keeping spiritually fit. Bodily exercise is all right, but spiritual exercise is much more important . . . because that will help you not only now in this life, but in the next life too."

I TIMOTHY 4:7-10 (TLB)

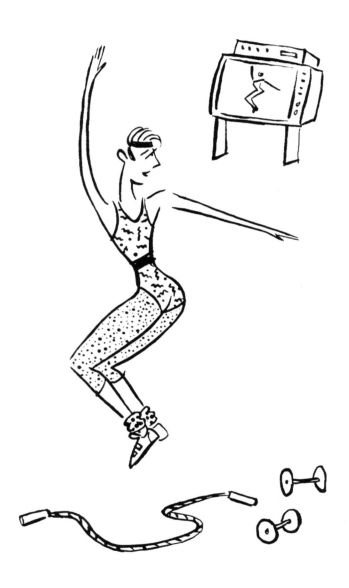

But I Hate to Exercise!

MAYBE YOU ARE ONE OF THOSE YOUNG women who pops out of bed at the crack of dawn, jumps into your leotards or jogging suit, and can't wait to start exercising. Pray for me, will you? For years I tried to psych myself into believing that I genuinely enjoyed exercising. Fat chance! Even though I knew physical exercise improved my appearance, energy level, health, and overall attitude, I could barely bring myself to put my body through the rigors of working out.

Calisthenics can build up the body. Courses of study can train the mind. But the real champion is the person whose heart can be educated.

FRED RUSSELL

P.E. was my least favorite class. To me, physical fitness wasn't much fun. Fortunately, the "no pain, no gain" approach to exercise is rapidly becoming a thing of the past. In fact, doctors now tell us that many of our everyday activities are actually exercise. From climbing stairs, making beds, and scrubbing floors, to washing the car, cleaning house, and walking the dog, every move you make burns calories.

Granted, some forms of exercise burn more calories than others. A 130 pound woman can burn ten calories per minute swimming, twelve calories per minute jogging, or six calories per minute riding a bike. Believe it or not, you even burn about one and a half calories per minute while eating! Now, that's what I call exercise!

TWO COMMON MISCONCEPTIONS

The first misconception regarding exercise is that thin girls don't really need to work out. Not so. Everybody, young or old, plump or thin, needs some sort of exercise in order to keep her heart healthy and limbs limber. Even those girls who want to gain a little weight will benefit from a regular exercise program.

The second misconception concerning exercise is, "If I exercise, I'm going to develop big, ugly muscles and look like a guy!" Again, not so. Aerobic exercises help you burn the layer of fat surrounding your muscles which causes your body to look leaner, but that doesn't mean you are bulking up.

Even working with weights, if done correctly, will firm up feminine muscles rather than cause them to bulge, unless you overdo it or take steroids, both of which I strongly caution you against. Besides, most female bodies do not produce enough of the male hormone, testosterone, required for real bulky muscles. Personally, I am not interested in any exercise program that is going to cause me to look or feel like a man. I love being a woman. I believe God created me to be feminine, and frankly, I want my exercise program to enhance my femininity, not detract from it.

WHY EXERCISE?

Here are just a few of the positive things a proper exercise program will do for you:

1. It will strengthen your heart (which is a muscle, too).
2. It will increase your blood circulation, which does wonders for your skin and hair.
3. It makes your bones more flexible. This may not seem important to you now, but as you get older, if you neglect exercise you won't be able to enjoy many of the simple, physical activities you do now.
4. Exercise helps make you firmer, reducing the amount of your body's flappy, flabby fat.
5. It can help relieve you of emotional stress, calming your nerves.
6. If you are overweight, a good exercise program can help you lose weight safely and keep the weight off permanently (assuming you continue with proper exercise and eating habits).
7. Exercise improves your digestion.
8. It helps you sleep better at night.
9. It increases your self-confidence.
10. It improves your energy level.
11. Did I mention that it improves your overall appearance? Well, it does!

You probably know that exercise is good for you, that it helps you beat the body blahs. The problem is

You are most in need of exercise when you don't have any time for it.
LLOYD CORY

Most middle-class Americans tend to worship their work, to work at their play, and to play at their worship.

GORDON DAHL

establishing a workable exercise program that doesn't require you to be an Olympic athlete to maintain. You want something relatively simple that you can start easily and stick with.

I'm convinced the best exercise plan is one in which you cross-train. Cross-training is a relatively new approach to exercising. It intermingles three specific areas of exercise: aerobic, nonaerobic or strengthening, and stretching. Don't let all that scare you. You needn't do all three types of exercise at once. Instead, one day you may do aerobics, the next you can do stretching exercises, and the next you might do some weight training.

AEROBIC AND NONAEROBIC: WHAT'S THE DIFFERENCE?

To get the best results from your exercise program, you need to understand why you are doing a particular type of exercise. For example, what's the difference between aerobic and nonaerobic exercise? Should I do one and not the other? Should I work with weights? What good does stretching do anyway? Actually, most fitness experts now agree that most of us need all three: aerobic, non-aerobic, and stretching exercises.

Aerobic means "with the presence of oxygen." Obviously human beings need oxygen for everything we do, but aerobic exercises are designed specifically to get your heart pumping faster and your lungs breathing heavier. When done correctly, aerobic exercises strengthen your heart and lungs as they pump blood and oxygen throughout your system. Aerobic exercises are also the best way to burn excess fat in your body.

Nonaerobic exercises, sometimes known simply as strengthening exercises, are designed to deal with an isolated part of your body, one area at a time, strengthening the muscles in that area. The goal is not really to burn fat, as you do in aerobics. In nonaerobic exercises, the goal is to strengthen and tone your muscles.

Some examples of nonaerobic exercises are weight training, calisthenics, and isometrics, all of which tone one area of your body at a time. Doing sit-ups, for example, is a nonaerobic, strengthening exercise. It will work wonders for your waist and abdominal muscles, but will do virtually nothing for your legs or upper body.

Stretching exercises are designed primarily for flexibility. They are fun, relaxing, and easy to do, and they help keep your body limber and pliable. Let's look at the three areas of cross-training more closely.

AEROBIC EXERCISES

To be considered aerobic, an exercise should get your heart working at sixty-five to eighty percent of its maximum ability. This is sometimes known as your heart's "training rate." For most teenagers, this rate is approximately 125 to 155 heartbeats per minute.

How can you tell how rapidly your heart is beating? Easy. You can check your pulse by placing your two middle fingers on the opposite wrist or on the side of your neck. Feel around until you find your pulse. Then count the beats for ten seconds and multiply by six, or you can count the beats for six secounds and add a zero. A normal pulse rate is 72 to 80 beats per minute when you are resting. The better shape your heart is in, the lower your resting heart rate will be.

For aerobic exercise to be effective, you must get your heart pumping at its training rate for at least twelve to fifteen minutes, nonstop. Should you quit in the middle of your aerobic workout, your heartbeat will slow down, and you will lose the benefits of aerobics. It is also

I have fought the good fight, I have finished the race, I have kept the faith. Now there is in store for me the crown of righteousness, which the Lord, the righteous judge, will award to me on that day.

II TIMOTHY 4:7, 8A

very dangerous to stop exercising when your heart is hard at work. The key to aerobic exercises is to do them without stopping. In other words, for your aerobic exercise program to work, you'll need to work, too. Then when you are near the end of your workout, you need to gradually slow your pace so your heart can return to its normal rate.

Of course, before you begin any exercise program, check with your doctor. Some people have specific conditions which may limit their exercise regimen. Better to find out about any potential problems before causing complications.

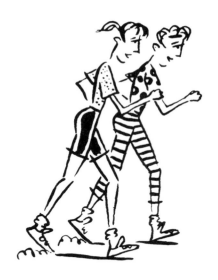

According to the exercise experts at the American College of Sports medicine, most of us "need a minimum of twenty to thirty minutes of aerobic activity three times a week to achieve and maintain cardiovascular fitness."[1] If you are just beginning an exercise program, plan to build your endurance gradually and consistently. Start by doing ten minutes of an aerobic activity three times a week. Each week add another five minutes up to thirty. That way you won't be tempted to give up. Many beginners quit before they've barely even started their exercise program because they have unrealistic expectations. They try to do too much, too soon, and they end up getting overly tired, sore, and discouraged. After a brief attempt at exercising, they give up in frustration.

A few examples of aerobic exercises are:

Brisk walking. Walking is great exercise; it works your heart and other muscles without straining or jolting your ankles, knees, and feet. Remember, though, you are trying to get your heart rate pumping. Casually walking in the park or cruising through the mall won't do it. You need to walk fast and continuously for about twenty minutes.

Jogging. Next to walking, jogging is one of the easiest but most effective exercises you can do. The toughest part about jogging is working up the desire to do it.

Before you begin, do some basic stretching exercises, some walking, or very slow jogging to limber up your calves and thigh muscles. Otherwise, you're just asking for soreness, aches, pains, and a plausible excuse for quitting your exercise program. Do some side bends and leg stretches, but go easy. Don't bounce, just stretch. These warmups aren't supposed to hurt. Also, keep breathing regularly. For some reason, many people tend to hold their breath for long periods of time while exercising. Don't do it. Muscles need oxygen to loosen up, so breathe as normally as possible, even though you may be a bit winded when you first begin your exercise regimen.

It's best to jog on grass or dirt if possible. Jogging on concrete or paved sidewalks and roads is hard on your legs and feet.

Take your time. Jogging rapidly will not really burn more calories than going slowly, so build endurance rather than speed. So what if your friends think you are moving in slow motion. At least you're doing something!

Some experts say you should jog for thirty minutes, three times per week. If that works for you, great! But don't overdo it. Find a pattern that you can enjoy. If you dread a lengthy jogging session, before long, you will probably give up jogging completely. Start slowly and build. Try ten or fifteen minutes for starters.

You can jog alone or in a group, inside or outside; the benefits are the same (although the fresh air you get jogging outdoors is good for you, too). If you are

Love is a great good that makes every heavy thing light. It is not burdened by the load it carries, and it sweetens the bitter.

THOMAS A KEMPIS

The most eminent graces turn to deadly poison if we rest on them in self-complacent security.

FRANCOIS FENELON
SPIRITUAL LETTERS TO WOMEN

jogging indoors and want to beat the boredom, try wearing or carrying a cassette player and listening to some Christian music while you jog.

Swimming. Swimming is a terrific all-round conditioning exercise. For an all-over workout, it's tough to beat. Keep in mind, though, we're talking about aerobic exercise here, not just lounging around the pool or checking out the guys at the beach. To be effective, you must swim nonstop for about fifteen minutes. Any stroke will do: sidestroke, breaststroke, doggie-paddle, or whatever. Just keep moving!

Jumping rope. I know this old favorite sounds like kid's stuff, but have you ever noticed how much energy those kids have? Jumping rope works wonders on your body. It really gets your heart pumping! You don't need to jump high, just high enough to clear the rope. Start with twenty jumps each day and gradually build up the number. One caution. Just because this exercise is simple, don't let it fool you. It can still cause extreme stiffness and soreness in your legs if you try to do too much or don't take the time to warm up before starting. Also, be sure to cool down after this or any exercise by walking and stretching when you are done.

Aerobic dancing. By dancing, I'm not talking about snuggling up to your best guy on a dimly lit dance floor. I'm referring to aerobic exercise dancing. A multitude of audio and videocassettes featuring structured exercise to music are now available. Your local Christian bookstore probably stocks many of these programs that include Christian music; I highly recommend them. That way you can exercise your body and nourish your spiritual life at the same time. If you prefer, make up your own routines to your favorite music. You'll need at least twenty minutes' worth of aerobic dancing to make it

It will not hurt you at all to consider yourself less righteous than others, but it will be disastrous for you to consider yourself better than even one person.

THOMAS A KEMPIS

beneficial to your heart and lungs.

Bike riding. My husband, Gary, and I love to ride our bikes! It's great fun and it's something we can do together. Again, you can't stop and start if you want the exercise to work. You've got to keep pedaling for a minimum of twenty minutes. No fair coasting!

Gary even bought me a wind-trainer, sort of a tripod platform, so I can use my bike as a stationary bike indoors when the weather is bad. It's not as much fun as cycling outdoors, but the exercise value is just the same.

Exercise machines. If you are a member of a health club, you probably have access to an assortment of fancy machinery to help you exercise. Machines such as Nautilus equipment and others are quite effective if used properly. On the other hand, beware of advertising scams on television and in magazines that promise instant body shaping, weight loss, or an easy, effortless path to physical perfection. Most of these "wonder machines" are rip-offs. I'm not saying they don't work; I'm just saying you don't need them. You can get the same results for free with a proper exercise program at home.

Step aerobics. A popular new form of aerobic exercise is step aerobics. This new workout is actually a variation on good, old-fashioned stair climbing, only nowadays, you can pick up your step and take it with you when you are done. Step aerobics is designed to improve cardiovascular endurance and tone and tighten the muscles in your buttocks and legs.

Most of us need encouragement to keep at our exercise program. You may have a good friend or a group with whom you can get together and exercise. It can be great fun, and you can help motivate each other. Unfortunately, because of the sporadic schedule I keep as a Christian artist who is on the road a lot, I've found

The less time one has, the more carefully it should be managed. If you wait for free, convenient seasons in which to fulfill real duties, you run the risk of waiting forever; especially in such a life as yours. No, make use of all chance moments. . . .
FRANCOIS FENELON, IN A LETTER TO A BUSY DUCHESS, 1689
SPIRITUAL LETTERS TO WOMEN

What does God require of you but simply to do the truth?

ELISABETH ELLIOT

NO GRAVEN IMAGE

that I need to squeeze my exercise sessions in wherever and whenever I can.

Consequently, I've become a big fan of exercise videos. The videos are great for me because I can exercise right at home. I'm not the type of person who will take the time to travel across town to work out in a gym, but in the privacy of my own TV room, at my convenience . . . okay, I can do that.

The instructional videos are also good for me because most of them have two workouts going on at the same time, one for beginners, the other for more advanced exercisers. I follow along with the one most comfortable for me. When I get really tired, I stop or take a break. That gives me a chance to work at my own pace without feeling embarrassed about going too fast or too slow, or feeling that I am holding someone else back.

The drawback to video workouts is obvious: the people on the screen keep doing the same thing every day! As such, it's easy to get bored unless you vary the videos you use or the part of the program you follow.

I prefer low-impact programs over high-impact ones. In low-impact exercises, you don't jump as high, kick as high, and in general, everything takes place closer to the floor. You always have at least one foot on the floor. For me, that helps prevent shin splints, a painful result of the muscles pulling away from the bone. It also is easier on knees and other joints that are jarred during higher impact aerobics.

I also like to work with weights, but I limit myself to using two-pound weights to strengthen my arms and upper-body areas. I once went to heavier weights and ended up having to go to a chiropractor to put my back into place. Since I am only toning and shaping my body, I'm not really interested in building up my muscles. As I said, I have no desire to be a female bodybuilder! Body-builders use heavier weights and do fewer repetitions. Using smaller weights and doing more repetitions builds endurance and works well for me.

NONAEROBIC, STRENGTHENING EXERCISES

With all the emphasis on aerobic exercise nowadays, it's easy to neglect nonaerobic, strengthening exercises. Granted, by doing aerobics you will burn fat and see an overall improvement in your appearance, but unless you do some strengthening exercises, you are still going to look and feel like a mushball.

Where should you start with your spot training? Anyplace you know that needs toning: stomach, hips, thighs, waist, arms, or buttocks. That about covers everything, doesn't it? Of course, if your stomach is in great shape but lately your thighs have been reminding you more and more of tree trunks, you need only do enough stomach exercises to keep your muscles toned. Go after those thighs, though, with a vengeance! As you trim down and tone up, you will be pleased to discover that by combining aerobics and a regular strengthening regimen, you can keep your body in excellent shape.

Most trainers suggest beginning with a minimum of fifteen to twenty minutes of strengthening and toning exercises at least twice a week. As with aerobics, begin slowly, with a shorter amount of time and fewer repetitions, and build from there.

Many women's magazines offer an assortment of strengthening and toning exercises, so I won't go into great detail here. Nevertheless, I do want to share with you a few of my secrets for dealing with some of the more obvious trouble spots.

But my eyes are fixed on you, O Sovereign Lord. . . . When my spirit grows faint within me, it is you who know my way.
PSALM 141:8; 142:3 (NIV)

How to Flatten Your Tummy

Although your stomach is one of the easiest places in which to gain weight, it is one of the toughest places to tighten. That's because your abdominal muscles get extremely little exercise through the normal course of your day, unless you purposely decide to exercise them.

For your lower abdominal muscles (often referred to simply as "lower abs"): Lie on your back with your hands tucked under your buttocks. Keeping your lower back flat on the floor, point your legs straight up in the air and cross them at your ankles. Now, while keeping your knees slightly bent, lift your hips toward the ceiling, exhaling as you do. Inhale as you bring your hips back down to the floor. Repeat ten times for beginners, twenty times maximum. (See drawing.)

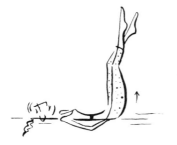

For your upper and middle abdominals: Lie on your back with your knees bent and your feet flat on the floor. Extend your arms and clasp your hands above your head. Then, starting with your back flat on the floor and your arms and hands extended, curl your upper body toward your knees as if attempting to do a sit-up, being sure to keep your lower back on the floor. Exhale as you curl up, then inhale as you allow your shoulders to come down to the floor again. Ten to twenty reps should do. (See drawing.)

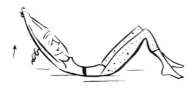

For another easy but effective stretching exercise for your stomach, get down in a push-up position, but keep your hips and knees on the floor. Now, push your upper body toward the ceiling without locking your elbows or moving your hips. Try this one five to ten times. That's enough! (See drawing.)

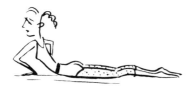

Of course, the old faithfuls, sit-ups and partial sit-ups, are great for your stomach muscles, too.

EXERCISING YOUR HIPS

Lie on your right side with your right leg slightly bent, right hand stretched out above your head. Now, cross your left leg over your right leg and raise your left leg about ten to twelve inches above your right leg. Hold it there for two counts; then, lower your left leg for two counts, but don't let it touch your right leg or the floor. Repeat ten times; then switch sides, working your right leg. (See drawing.)

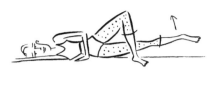

Another effective hip exercise: Lie on your back, with your arms extended, palms facing up. Bring your knees in close to your chest. Now, keep your knees together as you roll your legs all the way to the right until your hip touches the floor. Slowly, bring your legs back over your chest, then roll to the left until your opposite hip touches the floor. Keep your shoulders flat on the floor as you do ten to twenty repetitions. (See drawing.)

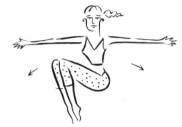

FIXING FLABBY ARMS

Start with some basic arm circles, rotating ten to twenty times in each direction every day. (See drawing.) Then, if you have some two-pound, hand-held weights (if you don't have weights, use a heavy book, a brick, or even some canned goods!), try this: Hold a weight in each hand and stand with your back straight, arms at your side. Make sure your knees are slightly bent and your feet are apart and squared with your shoulders. Now, slowly bring your weights straight up to shoulder level. Pause, then lift the weights all the way above your head. Hold for one count, then reverse the procedure, slowly bringing your weights back first to your shoulder level, then to the start position. Do several sets of ten. (See drawing.) These are great for your shoulder areas.

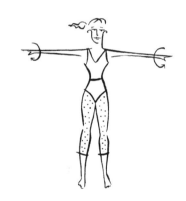

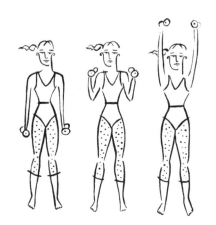

Basic curls with your weights will build your biceps.

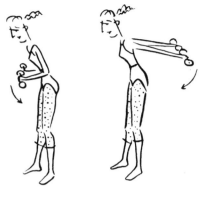

For your triceps, start from a standing position, feet about shoulder width apart, leaning slightly forward with your weights about waist high. Now, with your arms straight, bring the weights back until they are parallel with the line of your back. Hold for one count and return. (See drawing.) Several sets of ten, three times a week will tone your triceps.

THINNING THOSE THUNDER THIGHS

This is another area where flab loves to hang out, since your inner thighs rarely are exercised in your normal daily routines. One of the simplest, yet most effective thigh trimmers is the leg lift. Lie on your side, legs together and extended straight out. Now lift your top leg eighteen inches or so, with your knee and toe pointing forward, stretching your inner thigh muscle. Slowly lower your leg, but do not let it touch your bottom leg. Do ten repetitions, then roll over and repeat with your other leg. (See drawing.)

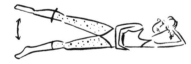

To tone your outer thighs, do the same exercise, but roll your hip forward so your toe and knee point toward the floor. (See drawing.) You'll feel this one in the back of your legs.

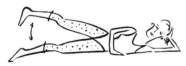

For another great thigh trimmer, for both inner and outer thighs, lie on your side again, propping yourself up with your forearm. (Be sure to keep your back straight—don't let it sag.) Keep both legs together, one on top of the other, and extended straight. Now, slowly lift then lower both legs. Turn over and reverse. This is a tough one, but it's worth it! Three sets of five should get you started. (See drawing.)

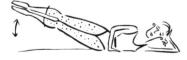

These are just a few examples of spot training and strengthening exercises. Many others are equally effective. Find a few that work for you, specific to each area of your body. Then incorporate the various exercises into your regimen as needed. Change your routine often so you don't get bored doing the same exercises all the time.

STRETCHING

The third prong in cross-training is stretching the muscles to keep them flexible and limber. For most of us, flexibility exercises can do an amazing amount of good. When your muscles are tense, they tend to cut off their own circulation, which often results in muscle aches and fatigue. Stretching can help relieve that.

Poor flexibility is also a leading culprit in lower back pain. The lower back muscles get stiff if they are not adequately stretched, and you begin to feel old before your time.

A good stretching session, done after an aerobic workout or a strengthening workout with weights, will ward off the next-day muscle soreness that often plagues people who are just beginning an exercise program.

Many people confuse stretching exercises with warming up before another type of exercise. You should always warm up before exercising, but the best way to do that is not prolonged stretching. In fact, stretching cold muscles could do more harm than good. Light stretches such as side bends or reaches are okay for warmups. Remember the old song, "Bend and stretch, reach for the stars"? But to really stretch your muscles, the best time to gain maximum flexibility is after a workout, before your cool-down time, while your muscles are still warm and pliant.

How should you stretch your muscles? Here's one example: Sit on the floor with one leg extended in front of you, the other leg bent back, right next to your body.

My goal is God himself . . . at any cost, by any road.
AMY CARMICHAEL

KOHILA

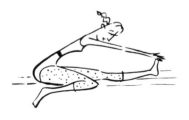

Now, lean as far over your extended leg as you can, keeping your back straight and your toes pointed up. Hold the stretch for at least ten seconds but no more than forty-five seconds. (See drawing.) When you begin to feel extreme discomfort, let go of the stretch. You don't want to tear the muscle, but usually if you hold a stretch long enough, you will feel your muscles begin to relax and give a little. Now reverse legs and do the same for your other side.

Whatever you do, don't bounce or jerk your muscles when stretching. Even when they are warm, muscle fibers can tear. Ligaments will, too. Again, easy does it. Stretching exercises should not be painful or uncomfortable.

One caution concerning stretching exercises: Some of the stretching programs advertised on television or in magazines include yoga, visualization, and other New Age types of "spiritual" overtones. For example, one well-known star of several extremely popular exercise videos, advocates the use of yoga, a practice derived from Hinduism. My advice? Avoid such programs. Plenty of great exercise videos are available that extol Christian values. You needn't expose yourself to the subtle, mind-controlling influences of Hinduism or other religions in order to stretch your muscles.

KIM'S TIPS FOR PROPER EXERCISE

1. Always warm up before doing any kind of exercise. You can warm up by walking, jogging slowly, or doing simple stretches. Two to four minutes of warmup is good; five to ten minutes is better.
2. Vary your exercise regimen to avoid boredom. Do different exercises each week that will work the same areas of your body.

3. If you are just beginning your exercise program, consult with your doctor; then start slowly and work up to longer time periods.

4. Try to do some form of exercise at least three or four days per week for twenty or thirty minutes. If you can work in more than that, great! It's good to give your body a rest, however, so it can repair sore or torn muscles. If you push yourself too much, you can end up with serious injuries.

5. Take advantage of everyday opportunities to exercise. Ride a bike or walk short distances rather than riding in a car. Take the steps instead of the elevator or escalator. Whatever you are doing that requires physical exertion, put a little more "oomph" into it.

6. Don't expect instant results from your exercise program, especially if you are hoping to lose weight. You didn't put on that extra weight overnight, and it won't come off overnight, either. If you go for the quick burn, you run the risk of burning out. Be patient, but also be persistent. Keep at it, and you can be assured of success.

7. Don't overdo it. In an interview, super-model Elle Macpherson revealed an interesting story about herself. She explained that her exercise regimen included forty-five minutes on a StairMaster, then forty-five minutes on a stationary bike, followed by forty-five minutes of running and weight work, plus an entire aerobics class and separate stretching session. Whew! I get tired just thinking about all that. So did Elle, apparently. She said, "I'd do 1,000 sit-ups each day and feel guilty if I wanted to stop at 900. My body didn't look any different and I was miserable. So I quit."

No, she didn't give up exercise altogether. She

I now realize, God, how much you have given me. So much that was beautiful and so much that was hard to bear. Yet whenever I showed myself ready to bear it, the hard was directly transformed into the beautiful.

ETTY HILLESUM, TWO MONTHS BEFORE DYING IN THE GAS CHAMBERS AT AUSCHWITZ QUOTED FROM *ETTY HILLESUM; AN INTERRUPTED LIFE*

still jogs, does some weight training, and does other exercises, too. But now, the moment she feels miserable, she stops.

The point is, don't attempt to do too much. If you feel fatigued, quit for today. It's better to do a little exercise than to give up and do none at all.

8. Keep in mind that the ultimate goal is to glorify God with our bodies (I Corinthians 6:20). The Bible says that your body is the temple of the Holy Spirit. It seems only right to me that we take care of God's property as best we can.

One of these days, though, our physical bodies will be dead and gone, nothing but dust in a box. But our relationship with Jesus Christ will last throughout eternity. That's why we want to constantly strive to cultivate those qualities of inner beauty such as peace, joy, and love that will last forever, those qualities that will cause others to be attracted to Him.

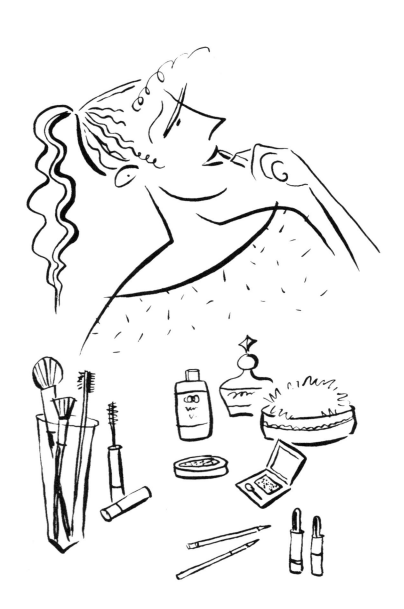

In Living
Color

MY FRIEND CARTER BRADLEY IS A professional makeup artist who has helped me with my makeup for several of my album covers. One of the best tips I've learned from Carter is realizing that the purpose of wearing makeup or using any cosmetics is not to hide the real you or even to cover the imperfections that we all have (though it does help). Makeup is meant to enhance your natural appearance, highlighting your best points and minimizing your weak areas.

155

It is futile to use makeup to alter your facial features in an effort to look like someone else. You can't do it, and why would you want to? God created you, with your unique characteristics. Ideally, makeup should be an added touch that brings out the best in your face, your features.

What I am eager for is that all the Christians there will be filled with love that comes from pure hearts, and that their minds will be clean and their faith strong.

I TIMOTHY 1:5 (TLB)

WHEN IS IT TIME TO START WEARING MAKEUP?

Some women never get into the whole idea of wearing makeup; they choose not to wear it, or at least not very much of it. They prefer a more natural look. Others have religious convictions about wearing makeup, although oftentimes, those convictions have been legalistically imposed rather than spiritually discerned from studying the Bible. Some women go way overboard in their use of makeup, giving themselves a painted-doll look. Many other women prefer to wear makeup, but still go for the most natural look possible.

There are no specific birthdays that serve as established bench marks, no signposts that say, "Okay, now you are old enough to wear makeup." Still, most parents prefer that their daughters wait until the mid-to-late junior high years before starting to wear makeup. Wearing makeup before then is usually an attempt by an immature young lady to look older and feel more grown up.

We've all seen the sorry paint jobs that some girls do on themselves, hoping to impress their peers (or worse still, the older guys). Usually these efforts leave more an impression of Bozo the Clown than anything else. That's why wearing makeup may have much more to do with maturity than it does with age. Don't begin until you really want to, your parents permit you, and you have a basic understanding of how to use makeup. Even then, don't allow your peers to pressure you into wearing makeup.

THE START OF SOMETHING GOOD

When you do begin to wear makeup, you'll want to create the best impression possible. Start by finding a place where you can apply your makeup in the light in which you are going to be seen—daylight. If you can, open the window shades to get as much natural light as possible. Makeup mirrors with bright lights are helpful but not absolutely necessary. Avoid fluorescent lights when putting on makeup. You won't be able to see the true colors under fluorescent light; then when you step outside into the daylight, your coloration will be off.

Also, before applying any makeup, be sure that your face is clean. Go through your normal cleansing routine, and don't forget to moisturize. Besides helping your skin maintain its natural moisture, this will also prepare your face for your foundation.

A SURE FOUNDATION

Speaking from just a beauty standpoint, not everyone needs to wear foundation. However, with the availability of foundations that include sunscreens and other products which actually protect your skin from the everyday effects of sun, pollution, and dirt, most experts agree that it is better for your skin if you do wear a foundation.

The primary purpose of using a makeup foundation is to create a base, even out your skin tone, give your face one overall color, and give your skin a smooth finish. What a foundation is not meant to do, or should

Make sure Jesus is your foundation for life. Without Him, everything else is ultimately a waste of time.

not do, is change your skin color or look as though you are wearing a mask. Today's makeup foundations are designed to be light and subtle, enhancing your skin tones.

The color of your foundation should match your natural skin color as closely as possible. You'll probably have to experiment with this. You may even have to combine two colors to get the one that is closest to your color. It is possible to have a foundation color blended specifically to match your skin color; this, however, can be expensive and is not usually necessary. Plan on spending an hour or two in the cosmetics section of your local department store or drugstore. Ask your mom to come along, or a close friend who will be absolutely honest with you, and don't be too shy to ask for her opinion.

Foundation makeup comes in several forms: liquid, cream, cake, powder, even a mousse. I recommend an oil-free, water-based foundation, especially during your teenage years. Oil-based foundations tend to be too heavy for teenage skin and promote acne. Liquids are the most easily used and can give you a light, subtle look.

To apply your foundation, pour a small dot of makeup onto your fingertip and start dotting it onto your nose, cheeks, chin, and forehead. (Be sure that your hair is pulled back, away from your face.) Then smooth and blend the makeup using your fingers or a small, damp sponge, working out from the center of your face toward your hairline, but be very careful not to push the foundation too far into your hair. Blend the makeup down onto your throat, underneath your jaw, and fade the foundation into your neck. You don't need to coat your neck, just allow the makeup to gently blend into it.

Use smooth, light strokes to smooth out your

foundation. Never pull or stretch your skin. The idea of foundation, remember, is to give your face one continuous color, so be careful not to streak it by rubbing. Put on a little bit at a time and blend it into your skin. You're not painting a house here; you should be able to see your skin peeking through the makeup. Be sure to blend over the chin, right up to your ears, and as close to your hairline as you can get.

As I said, many young women don't even need foundation. If you are one of the lucky ones, you can get the same effect by simply brushing on a light layer of powder that is similar to your natural skin tone.

POWDER POWER

The purpose of applying powder is to set your makeup in place. Powder also absorbs any excess oil lying on your skin. It gives your face a nice, smoothed-out effect.

Powder can be bought in two forms—loose, which is translucent (meaning it has a good light-reflecting quality) and can be applied directly from the container with a large brush; or pressed, which is what is put in compacts to carry with you in your purse for quick touch-ups throughout the day.

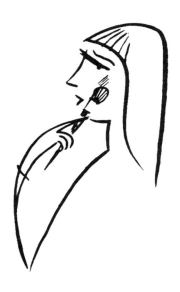

Some women prefer colored powders, but I prefer a color close to my actual skin color. The lightest, most transparent powder I can get, the closer to my actual skin color (which is light), the better.

Don't rub the powder into your skin. If you do, you will remove the makeup beneath and your face will look streaked. Instead, apply it gently over your face, then brush off the excess with a brush, puff pad, or cotton ball. A brush works best. Be especially careful around your eyes.

Isn't it odd? We often blush about what we should boast about, and we boast about what we should blush about.

Let your eyes look straight ahead, fix your gaze directly before you. Make level paths for your feet and take only ways that are firm.

PROVERBS 4:25, 26 (NIV)

BEAUTIFUL BLUSHES

An appropriate blusher is probably one of the most useful of all your colored cosmetics. A blusher can bring warmth, glow, and a healthy look to your face. Although blushers come in creams, sticks, or liquids, I think the easiest to use is powder.

Blush gets its name because of the effect it simulates on your face. When you blush because you have been embarrassed or surprised, blood rises to the surface in your cheeks, creating a rosy color. That is the idea behind makeup known as blush. It is intended to create that same sort of look (without the embarrassment, hopefully). Keep that in mind as you brush on your blush and you will know exactly where to apply it: the same areas that fill with color when you blush naturally—your cheeks, chin, and the top edges of your forehead. Some people redden in their necks when they blush, but that's not the best place to wear blush if you're wearing a blouse with a collar or a high-necked dress.

DO YOU SEE WHAT I SEE?

Your eyes are the focus of your face. Often they are the part of you other people notice first. Frequently, the first impression you make has a lot to do with the way your eyes look. So let's make them look the best we can!

To make their eyes look great, many women use three types of makeup: eye shadow, eyeliner (or pencil), and mascara. My preference is to use all three, but not all women do. Experiment and find what works for you.

STRIKING SHADOWS

The purpose of eye shadow is to brighten your eyes by slightly coloring the area around them. Remember, we are trying to highlight your eyes, not the surrounding area. As such, you'll probably want to use a neutral to beige or gray shadow, not bright green, fluorescent orange, blue, or lavender. Those colors may look great on the girls in the magazines, but at school or work, they can make you look like a clown. Also, unless you are doing a mime show, stay away from white. If you use white eye shadow, your eyes will look like something between a raccoon and an owl!

The most frequent mistake beginners make when it comes to eye makeup is that they draw attention to their makeup rather than to their eyes. The best eye makeup is subtle; you hardly notice it is there, but you'd sure notice if it weren't! Picking a color that really works for you is half the battle. Here's a tip: Choose shadow shades that will complement your eyes, not match your wardrobe!

Bright eyes gladden the heart.
PROVERBS 15:30

Eye shadow comes in several forms—the most popular are grease-based creams or powders. Pressed-powder shadows are the easiest to use and are my preference. Most come with their own brush or sponge-tipped applicator, but a soft "artist's" brush about one quarter inch wide will give you better control. You can purchase these brushes at most makeup counters, or for the "real thing," stop by an art supply shop.

If you use powder-based eye makeup, apply your foundation and powder to your eyelid before putting on any eye shadow. If you use a grease-based makeup, apply powder after you do your eyes so the makeup will set. Then apply your shadow over the lid, starting from the inner corner and working toward the center of your eyelid. Blend the shadow out toward the edge of your eye and upward toward your eyebrows.

ILLUMINATING LINES

Eyeliners are used to line the eyes right at the base of your eyelashes. Lining makes your eyelashes look fuller and your eyes more defined. Use a soft eyeliner pencil to line your eyelids from the inside corner to the outer edges. As you line your lids, gently try to color the lid in between each eyelash. Then when you have gone all around your eye, very gently smudge the lines you have just drawn, using a soft cotton swab or Q-Tip. This smudging gives your eyes a more natural look, rather than looking as though someone painted a ring around your eyelids. Some women line the inside of their lower eyelids with a white pencil for a bolder effect, but I don't think it's really necessary or sanitary.

As with your eye shadow, choose an eyeliner color that can coexist with your eyelashes. Although some girls will line their eyelids with outlandish colors, a more natural look can be achieved by using black, brown, gray, or charcoal eyeliner.

MAGNIFICENT MASCARA

Mascara, too, comes in a multitude of colors, but a black or brown mascara usually works best, unless your hair is blonde. If so, you may want to use a lighter mascara. In years past, a woman with blonde hair would not wear dark mascara because it was a dead giveaway that she was a "bottle blonde"—someone who had dyed her hair. Nowadays, most stigmas about hair coloring have fallen by the wayside, so you will sometimes see blondes wearing extremely dark mascara on their lashes. It is an acceptable look right now, but don't be surprised if the trend goes back to lighter lashes for fair-haired women.

Be very careful not to drip or smear mascara anywhere on your face. It is a real pain to get off without messing up the makeup you just put on. If you do smear some, use a wet Q-Tip to get it off. Don't rub.

A good mascara application really brings your eyes to life, so apply it carefully. Put on a thin coat, starting with the upper lashes. Many young women who are inexperienced with mascara seem to think more is better, so they just glob it on in a hurry. Wrong! Several thin coats will look much better than one heavy mess. Between each coat, use an eyelash brush or comb to gently separate each lash, making sure that none are left sticking together. To help prevent lashes from sticking, be sure to allow the mascara to dry between applications.

One reminder about mascara: Unless you use a waterproof type, it will run when it gets wet. If you will be swimming, sweating, or crying over the latest tear-jerking book or movie, you better go with waterproof mascara or carry plenty of tissue with you. Be careful, though. You can seriously damage your eyes should you get any waterproof mascara in them. To safely remove waterproof mascara, use an oil-free eye makeup remover designed specifically for that purpose.

One other word of warning regarding mascara: Never share your mascara with anyone else, and never use someone else's mascara. It is extremely unsanitary and an easy way to pass bacteria that causes eye infections. It is unwise to borrow someone else's makeup of any kind, but especially avoid sharing mascara.

EXPRESSIVE EYEBROWS

In addition to eye shadow, liner, and mascara, some women add color to their eyebrows. For most teenagers it is really not necessary, but if you feel it is, use a powder or an eyebrow pencil the same color as your brows and lightly draw short, soft lines to fill in your eyebrows.

Don't draw one long line. You'll look like your three-year-old brother got after you with his crayons! Think as if you are drawing in individual hairs. Notice the length of the hairs on your eyebrow and try to match them with your pencil. Never try to change the color of your eyebrows with a powder or pencil. It will just look silly. The best way to change the color of your eyebrows is to dye them, but relatively few women find eyebrow dying necessary to look attractive.

Your eyebrows should follow a natural line to match your face shape. Today, the easiest way for many women to alter their face shape is by changing the thickness of their brows. If done correctly, this can enhance your look; if it's done poorly, the results can be disastrous. In most cases, you will only need to remove stray hairs from the bottom of your brow or thin out overly thick brows.

I'm all for shaping your eyebrows if they need it, but don't grab your tweezers and start plucking hairs at random. Before becoming a "mad tweezer," try brushing your eyebrows. You may not need as much hair removal as you think. Constant plucking could cause your eyebrow hairs not to grow back, so don't pluck more than necessary. If you must pluck, the best time is after a shower or after you have thoroughly washed your face.

I gaze into her shining eyes,
With joy my soul transcends;
And yet—I wonder is it love
Or shiny contact lens?
SHELBY FRIEDMAN

LIP SERVICE

Like your eyes, proper lip service can make or break your makeup look. Whether you play them up or keep a more subtle look, your lips will tell a lot about you.

As with other makeup, you can choose from an array of colors for your lips—every color imaginable is showing up on lips nowadays, often more for shock effect than aesthetic value. But unless you want to look like a reject from a heavy metal band audition, I'd stay with more natural colors.

Besides, the range of more natural colors available between light peach and dark burgundy is astounding! Consequently, many women collect lipstick more than any other cosmetic. You may want to match your lipstick color to your mood or the occasion, from bright and sassy to calm and subdued.

As a general rule, you'll find that the colors that work well for you are the same ones you have chosen in your favorite dress-up clothes. For example, if you rarely wear clothes with deep burgundy, chances are that a lipstick with deep burgundy tones will not be your choice either.

There are no hard and fast guides, so you needn't be afraid to experiment. Just think of what colors of lips you've seen, and you'll have some broad parameters. Also, keep in mind the colors you have already used in your makeup. Pick lipstick colors that will mesh with your natural colors, your clothing, and your makeup.

Lipsticks come in many forms—regular lipstick in a tube, lip color in a compact, color in tiny bottles, lipstick in wands, and lipstick in pencils. Thinner pencils with a slightly harder, waxy, formula are used to outline the lips in a slightly darker color. Use whatever works well for you.

Always use lipsticks that contain moisturizer to avoid drying or staining your lips. Your lips are constantly exposed to the elements and can easily become chapped, rough, dry, or cracked from lack of moisture. To help prevent this, during the day use lipsticks with moisturizer, and at night spread a dot of petroleum jelly on your lips before you go to bed. Lipsticks that contain sunscreen are also available. Not a bad idea, especially if you spend a lot of time outdoors.

Truthful lips will be established forever, but a lying tongue is only for a moment.
PROVERBS 12:19

Take your time when you are putting on your lip color, even if you are doing so between classes at school. Sloppy lipstick application will spoil the entire look you have been trying to create. If you don't have time to do it right, you may be better off wearing just a bit of lip gloss. Some women who don't care for colored lips but want a little protection from the elements wear only colorless lip gloss all the time.

My friend Carter tells me that professional makeup artists spend more time preparing a mouth than any other part of the face. If you rush when applying your lipstick, not only will you not get the desired result, but you will also destroy the positive effect created by the rest of your makeup.

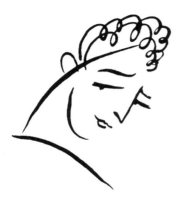

When you apply your other makeup, put some moisturizer, foundation, and light powder over the lips. If you want to line your lips, carefully use a lip pencil to trace the existing edge of your lips. Many women omit this step because of time, but it does add distinct definition to your lips.

Now you are ready to apply your lipstick. Using a tube or brush, carefully stroke on the color, starting with the center of the top lip and working out to the sides. Then do the lower lip the same way. When you are done, fold a clean tissue in half, hold it softly against your lips, and press gently with your fingertips. This blots the lipstick and helps it to set. Lift the tissue off slowly— don't pull or rub—from one side to the other.

There you go! With a little practice, you'll be able to do your entire regimen in ten to fifteen minutes. Honest! Sure, there will be special occasions when you may want to add highlights, while on the other hand, there will be days you may want to do a quick dash of blush, powder, and mascara and get out the door. Fine! Make your makeup work for you. Don't allow yourself to become a slave to your makeup. Keep it light. Keep it natural. Keep it you.

One other caution: Please do not apply your makeup in public. If you need a touch-up, do it in the rest room or a private area.

And most of all, don't forget that when the day is done, the makeup comes off! All of it. Never go to bed with your makeup still on your face.

INEXPENSIVE ISN'T CHEAP

When it comes to makeup, a higher price tag does not necessarily mean a better product. In fact, I am not in favor of expensive makeup products at all. If you're going to spend the extra money, invest in better skin-care and hair-care products. Sure, you should buy quality products, but ordinarily less-expensive makeup will do the trick just as well as the higher-priced brands.

The Master Designer created your natural colors to work well together—your hair, eyes, and complexion. All of our makeup efforts are merely enhancing the great job He has already done.

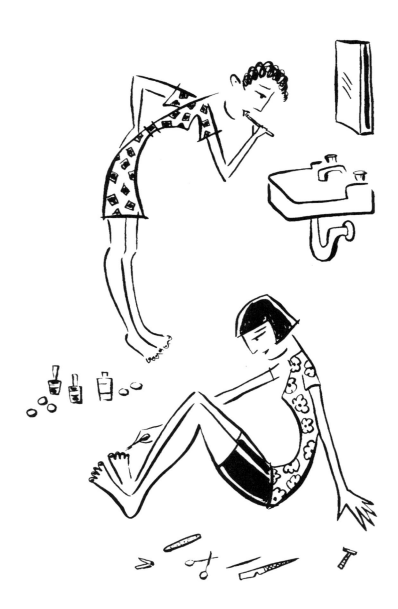

Special Effects

SALLY IS GORGEOUS. SHE HAS SHIMMERING, shining blonde hair, her makeup is meticulously applied, and her big, blue eyes sparkle with enthusiasm. She is in terrific physical shape, a beautiful picture . . . until she opens her mouth. Then, horror of horrors! Her teeth are awful.

So many people—fantastic, wonderful, beautiful, unique creations of God— are locked within themselves, peeping out longingly through curtained windows. O Father, O Father God, show me—show us—how to love ourselves properly and then to love others as we love ourselves.

KAY ARTHUR

TEACH ME HOW TO LIVE

TAKE CARE OF YOUR TEETH!

Taking care of your teeth is not a beauty option; it is a health essential! Unfortunately, many young women suffer severe tooth decay and gum disease simply because of neglect. They don't brush their teeth often enough, they rarely have a dental checkup, and some don't even own a container of dental floss!

Your teeth are one of your most valuable assets, and I'm not just talking about eating. A warm, friendly smile that reveals sparkling clean teeth does wonders for your appearance. On the other hand, when you know your teeth are full of gunk and your breath could knock over a bear at forty paces, smiling is no fun. Both problems are frequently the result of poor dental hygiene.

For starters, you can help prevent tooth decay by doing two simple things—cut down on sugar in your diet and correctly brush your teeth every day. Sugar is the biggest culprit when it comes to tooth decay. Along with the bacteria in plaque, the sticky substance that coats your teeth throughout the day, sugar creates a breeding ground for more bacteria, which continues to multiply and forms an acid in your mouth. This acid then attacks your tooth enamel. If the attack is allowed to continue (by your lack of brushing and flossing), the acid penetrates the enamel, spreads out into your tooth, and you end up with a cavity. By cutting down on your sugar intake, you can cut this attack off at the pass—your mouth!

Even with less sugar intake, to have healthy teeth and fresh breath you must remove the plaque from your teeth. That's where regular brushing and flossing can really make a difference.

Use a soft or medium bristle toothbrush that has tightly packed nylon tufts. When the tufts on the brush begin to look bent, it's time for a new brush. Brush at least twice a day, after every meal is even better, and never use anyone else's toothbrush!

Use a good toothpaste that contains fluoride. The toothpaste's mild abrasive quality helps to strip the plaque off your teeth, and the fluoride helps prevent cavities. I don't recommend using abrasive smokers' toothpastes to remove stains. They can damage your tooth enamel. If you have stains from soft drinks, coffee, or tea, talk to your dentist about the best way to get rid of them.

Speaking of smoking, I think it is one of the most disgusting habits a person can have. Talk about a turnoff! Besides messing up your lungs, smoking tends to create ugly yellow stains on your teeth. The smoke hangs in your hair and on your clothes like a sour-smelling mosquito net, and it makes your breath smell like something that should have been put in the trash weeks ago. Smoking isn't cool; it's stupid.

"Will smoking cause me to go to hell?"
"I don't know, but it will make you smell like you've been there!"

Flossing between your teeth is another good way to get plaque out of your mouth. With floss, you can get those hard-to-reach, in-between spots you can't reach with a toothbrush. It may take a little more time, but your teeth will thank you.

If you begin to floss regularly, your friends may thank you too. Many people with horrible breath could rid their mouths of the foul aromas by simply flossing their teeth. Some mouth odors are caused by the food you eat. That's unavoidable unless you avoid those foods. But when food particles become lodged between your teeth, odor is inevitable. Tooth decay, gum disease, abscesses, and other mouth infections can also cause bad breath. These sources of halitosis can be remedied at your dentist's office. Brushing, flossing, and professional cleaning all help.

Plan an appointment with your dentist once every six months, whether you have any cavities or not. It never hurts to check. Also, the professional cleaning you'll get from the dentist or dental hygienist will help prevent any future cavities.

If you want to see if you are brushing correctly and adequately, ask your dentist for some disclosing tablets. These are vegetable dyes you can dissolve in your mouth. The dye will stick to any leftover, decay-causing plaque. All you need to do then is rebrush your teeth removing all the dye-highlighted areas and the plaque at the same time.

Much work is also being done in the field of cosmetic dentistry. Nowadays, that million-dollar smile is possible, for a few dollars less. It still costs plenty of money, but crooked or protruding teeth can be straightened, stained or otherwise discolored teeth can be bleached or "painted," chipped teeth can be filed so the edges are even, and even extra space between teeth can be corrected—all for a price, of course.

Don't be duped by some of the dental whiteners offered on late-night television commercials. Instead, check with a reputable orthodontist, or several, before having dental work of this type done.

What if there were "disclosing tablets" for our spiritual lives, to reveal any "leftover sin"? Guess what? There are! In the Bible, they are known as the Ten Commandments.

HANDS AND NAILS

Have you ever seen a woman hide her hands in her pockets or under the desk or table? How sad, especially when caring for your hands is so simple. Granted, your hands probably take a beating. They're out there in all sorts of weather, getting banged around at school or work, diving into detergents and who knows what other chemical solutions. Sometimes, I just look at my hands and want to apologize for all the nasty ways I've treated them!

Your hands need as much care and attention as your complexion, but most of us don't do them justice. Here are some handy hints that will help:

1. Protect your hands as much as possible. Someone has said that you shouldn't put your hands anywhere you wouldn't put your face. That sounds nice but is totally unrealistic for most of us.
2. Always wear gloves outdoors in cold weather.
3. When you are working indoors, washing dishes, scrubbing floors, or cleaning the bathroom, wear rubber gloves.
4. Use a moisturizing hand cream as often as possible. Keep some near your sink or work area and reapply the cream every time you wash and dry your hands. Be sure to do the backs of your hands as well as the palms.
5. Make a few simple hand exercises a regular part of your day. Simply stretch your arms out, make a fist, then fling your fingers outward a few times. It will help keep your hands supple and reduce soreness.

Of course, one of the areas that most people notice about your hands is your fingernails. Nails needn't be long to be pretty, but they do need to be clean and well-manicured.

Some people are naturally blessed with strong, healthy nails. Others have difficulty growing long nails, or their nails crack, chip, or break often. I can identify. For most of my life, I've had really weak, short nails. Only in the past few years have my nails improved. I attribute the healthy nails to two things. One, I began taking vitamins, and two, I began a strict system of nail care. I've never liked the long "dagger-lady" look in nails, (although they were a "must" in my beauty pageant days), but now I can have medium-length, strong fingernails.

St. Augustine wrote: "God gives where he finds empty hands."
What does that imply to you?

*There are six things the
Lord hates, seven that are
detestable to him:
haughty eyes,
a lying tongue,
hands that shed
innocent blood,
a heart that devises
wicked schemes,
feet that are quick to
rush into evil,
a false witness who
pours out lies
and a man who stirs up
dissension among brothers.*
PROVERBS 6:16-19 (NIV)

As with most aspects of our external beauty regimen, you can pay a lot of money to have a professional give you a manicure, or you can do it at home for a few dollars' worth of materials and half an hour of your time. If you can afford it, it is fun to have your nails done professionally. Consider it an educational expense! Watch carefully what the manicurist does, then incorporate those ideas into your regimen at home. Here are a few ideas that have worked for me.

Collect the things you will need: a small bowl of warm water (a sponge in the water feels nice to press on), an emery board or nail file, an "orange stick" with cotton wrapped around it to remove excess polish from the nail, nail clippers (never cut your nails with regular scissors), nail polish remover, cuticle cream and cuticle remover, hand cream, and nail polish (including a base coat and a hardener). Now, put on some music and you're ready to begin!

1. Remove all of your old nail polish if you are wearing any. You can do this by wetting a cotton ball or tissue with nail polish remover. Press it onto your nail for just a few seconds, then wipe it off. The old polish will come right off. To remove polish from the edges of your nails, use a cotton swab soaked in remover.

2. Shape your nails by filing from the side of the nail toward the center. Don't make them too pointed. Pointed nails are weaker and tend to break more easily. Oval nails are stronger and more practical. File in one direction only, from the side to the tip, not back and forth.

3. Massage a dot of cuticle cream onto each nail's cuticle and dip your fingers into the bowl of soapy water for two to five minutes. Relax. Close your eyes and listen to music. (You could also use this time to

pray!) After dabbing your hands dry, take your orange stick, wrapped in a cotton tip, and gently push back the cuticle on each finger toward your knuckle. Never cut or tear your cuticle. It is there to protect the base of your fingernail. Rinse nails thoroughly before applying polish.

4. Apply a colorless base coat of polish to your nails. Allow it to dry. Some women prefer to wear only a base coat during the day. If you don't like colored nails, use two or three coats of clear polish to protect your nails. If you decide to go with a colored polish, try to think ahead to what you will be wearing, what activities you have coming up, and what sort of makeup you will be wearing. Choose a nail color that will work with your other colors. Your nail polish doesn't have to match your lipstick or other makeup, but it shouldn't clash with it, either. Basically, darker colors are more noticeable, but they also make your nails look smaller and show chips more easily.

5. Next, apply one coat of colored polish. Starting with the little finger, paint a semicircle of polish close to the cuticle, leaving a hair's width between the polish and the cuticle. Then paint the center of the nail and each side. Most polishes work best with two coats. Allow each coat to dry thoroughly (about five minutes) before going on to the next. Otherwise, your polish will chip.

6. Use your orange stick dipped in polish remover to carefully remove any excess polish around the nail.

7. Put a layer of sealer (colorless, clear polish) over your painted nails. This will harden the surface and hold the gloss. Brush a bit under the front of your nails, too.

Some girls say, "That all sounds like so much hassle just to have pretty fingernails. I'll just go to the store and buy some fake nails." I've done that. I've tried them all—press-on nails, glued-on nails, sculptured nails. When it comes to nails, if you can name it, I've probably tried it. Unfortunately, fake nails all have one major drawback: they tend to pop off at the most embarrassing moments. . . . Believe me, when you're talking nails, nothing beats your own.

If you have weak nails, try changing your diet a little. Vitamin B helps. It is in foods such as green beans and other green vegetables. Oh, it's in liver, too. Maybe you'll want to take a vitamin supplement, huh?

Naturally you will want to avoid biting your fingernails, a habit that not only creates horribly unsightly nails, but could crack a tooth, as well. And try not to use your nails as a hammer claw to pull staples or tacks out of your bulletin board. With a little common sense, your manicured nails will stay strong, healthy, and beautiful.

For one extra-special hand treatment, just before going to bed, mix a drop or two of peppermint oil (it's available at the grocery store in the baking section) with a bit of hand lotion. Apply generously to your hands, especially around your cuticles. Put on a pair of cotton gloves and sleep with them on. You'll be amazed at how soft your hands will feel in the morning!

FABULOUS FEET AND TWINKLING TOES

If you are like me, you probably only think about your feet when they hurt. I rarely think of my feet, and I certainly don't give much thought to other people's pedicure. Yet our feet are exposed for everyone to see

Everybody can be great. Because everybody can serve. You don't have to have a college degree to serve. You don't have to make your subject and verb agree to serve. You don't have to know Einstein's theory of relativity to serve. You don't have to know the second theory of thermodynamics in physics to serve. You only need a heart full of grace. A soul generated by love.

DR. MARTIN LUTHER KING JR.
QUOTED IN *AN UNFADING VISION*

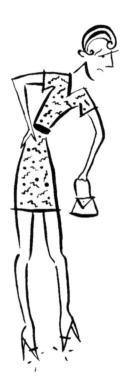

more often than we realize. If you wear open-toed shoes,
sandals, or spend much time at a pool or beach in the
summer, your feet are on display.

I doubt that we will ever spend as much time caring
for our feet as we do our faces, but it does seem unfair to
neglect them when they do so much for us. Here are a
few tips to help keep your feet user-friendly:

1. *Wear comfortable shoes.* When you are exercising,
   wear good quality shoes. You don't need to spend a
   fortune for a fancy name-brand shoe, but make sure
   your shoes give your feet, arches, and ankles good
   support. Always wear socks with your sport or
   exercise shoes.

   If you wear sneakers a lot, you're better off
   buying leather shoes with rubber soles. They will
   cost more, but the leather will allow your feet to
   "breathe" more than canvas shoes. Either way, be
   sure to let your sneakers air out after wearing, and
   wash your feet thoroughly. We always hear jokes
   about the guys' smelly sneakers, but you and I know
   they aren't the only ones whose feet sweat. There's
   nothing feminine about foot odor.

   I hate to say this, but high heels are awful for
   your feet. I'm not leading a crusade for flats (I'm
   only five foot, four inches tall myself!), but besides
   creating poor posture and other back problems, high
   heels cause many women to have intense soreness in
   their hamstring muscles and calluses on their feet.
   You'll probably wear them sometimes, especially for
   special occasions, but opt for lower shoes whenever
   you can.

2. *Massage your feet frequently.* Right after you take off
   your shoes is the best time. Besides being relaxing, a
   foot massage will revitalize your aching muscles.

How beautiful on the mountains are the feet of those who bring good news, who proclaim peace, who bring good tidings, who proclaim salvation.

ISAIAH 52:7

Have you ever thought your feet were beautiful? Why are these feet beautiful?

The troublesome thing about life is not that it is rational or irrational, but that it is almost rational.

G. K. CHESTERTON

During the day, kick off your shoes whenever possible. Flex your feet, point your toes, wriggle your ankles, or try picking up a pencil or some other small object with your toes. Hey, it beats daydreaming when your class gets boring!

3. *When you take a bath, be sure to scrub your feet.* Use a pumice stone or a loofah to strip off dead cells, and don't forget the bottoms of your feet.

4. *Moisturize, moisturize, moisturize!* Your feet deserve a little pampering, so pour on the body lotion.

5. *Give yourself a pedicure whenever possible.* The routine is basically the same as the manicure, except you will need a large bowl or basin in which to soak your feet. Ahhh, it feels so good!

REMOVING UNWANTED HAIR. OUCH!

God gave us fur on our bodies for a reason, but growing up in Florida, I often wondered why He gave us so much, especially since He knew we were going to spend so much time getting rid of it! Most women in our culture shave their legs and underarms. You probably will, too.

When you shave, you can use an electric razor or a safety razor. Most everyone but the people who make and sell electric razors will tell you that a safety razor will do a better job. It's all a matter of opinion. If you use a safety razor, you can shave in the tub or shower, using a sharp blade. Never use a dull blade; that's a sure way to shred your delicate skin. Many women simply use soapsuds to prepare the hair for removal, but if you have lots of hair, a shaving cream with a skin conditioner in it works wonders. If you are shaving the sensitive skin around your swimsuit lines, try applying some baby oil before and after shaving. Always shave against the direction your hair is growing.

Besides shaving, several other treatments will remove unwanted hair. The good news is they work; the bad news is they hurt and can be expensive.

Waxing. Waxing away unwanted hair is a beauty trick that has been around for ages. It is one of the best methods to remove hair on your upper lip, eyebrows, or chin. Never shave the hair on your face—unless you want to look like Grizzly Adams, that is. Nubs on your legs are tough enough to deal with; you don't need nubs on your face, too.

Waxing will usually take care of those stray hairs. There are two types of wax procedures available, hot wax and cold. Both are smoothed on in the direction your hair is growing, and then pulled off in the opposite direction. The first time you ever have your skin waxed, it would be wise to have it done professionally. Watch and learn before trying it yourself. If you do try it at home, be extremely careful! You can literally rip the skin off your face. Follow the manufacturer's directions explicitly.

Although the results of waxing are usually successful, the experience is not pleasant and your skin could possibly be irritated afterward. The good news is that the effects of waxing last longer than most other temporary hair-removal remedies. The bad news is that the hair will grow back in a few weeks.

Cream Depilatories. This is another form of hair removal that works but might be unpleasant. Depilatories actually use chemicals to dissolve the unwanted hair. The disadvantage is fairly obvious: any chemical strong enough to dissolve hair (think of Draino in your sink!) may also irritate your skin. Most depilatories are not to be used on your face. Facial skin is

I am just an ordinary looking woman who, like most women, has had to skillfully decorate her exterior! Physically, I'm not anything special. And that is what God wanted in order to accomplish His particular purpose in and through me. I bow to it; I bow to Him. I do the very best I can with what I have, and then I forget it.

KAY ARTHUR

TEACH ME HOW TO LIVE

far too sensitive for this sort of chemical treatment.

Electrolysis. This is a relatively new method of hair removal that has been proven effective. It is the closest thing we have to permanent hair removal, but the process is not fun. A fine wire is placed into the hair follicle down to its root. (Yes, this must be done for each hair!) Then a high frequency electric current—sort of FM for your follicles—is run down the wire. This severely damages or destroys the root, allowing the hair to be removed without pulling. In theory, the hair should never grow back, but if the process is not done correctly, it can.

Electrolysis (or diathermy) can be painful. Each hair removal feels like a hot pin has pricked your skin. It will take several trips to a professional treatment center or salon, which can really be expensive.

Pluck, pluck, pluck! Good, old-fashioned tweezers are still the safest and easiest method of getting rid of a relatively small amount of unwanted hairs such as stray eyebrow hairs. Although it is temporary, it does work. For best results (and the least ouch-factor!), apply a warm washcloth to the area you're going to pluck before pulling out the hair. Afterward, you may want to apply an antiseptic to guard against infection and to promote healing or an astringent to soothe the skin where the hair was removed.

Bleaching. Many women have a slight moustache above the upper lip. For some women, this hair is light, thin, and hardly noticeable; for others, it can be embarrassingly dark and full. Don't shave this hair! It will only grow back thicker. Bleaching is the best solution if you choose not to use one of the remedies I mentioned above.

Bleaching this hair has two advantages: it lightens the

hair, and because of the harsh action of the bleach, it often damages the hair shaft enough that it will not grow back or grows back very slowly. Bleaches can be bought at most beauty salons, but be sure the product is designed for facial hair. Even then, run a patch test on a portion of your skin to make sure you do not have an adverse reaction to the bleach. As always, if you experience any irritation or breakout, get rid of that product!

INTIMATE DETAILS

It would be a shame to spend all the time, effort, and money to present the best you possible, and then blow it by neglecting your basic feminine hygiene. Regular baths or showers, clean undergarments, feminine hygiene products, and deodorants are all part of intimately caring for your body.

Have you ever seen a physically attractive person who looks terribly lonely? Why is that?

Especially during your teenage years, your body is going through a lot of changes. Just keeping yourself clean and comfortable will do wonders for your self-confidence and help you to be more successful at making and keeping new friends.

But keep in mind that a squeaky clean body and a beautiful exterior can't conceal ugliness on the inside of a person. Jesus said, "From within, out of the heart . . . proceed the evil thoughts, fornications, thefts, murders, adulteries, deeds of coveting and wickedness, as well as deceit, sensuality, envy, slander, pride and foolishness" (Mark 7:21, 22). The most beautiful women in the world will still be lonely if they don't have inner beauty.

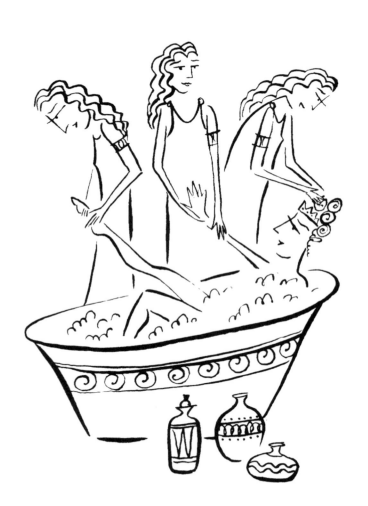

It's a Beautiful Life!

I F YOU HAVE NEVER READ THE STORY OF Esther in your Bible, you are missing a treat. It has more excitement and intrigue than the best mini-series on TV. It's all about sex, money, power, and double crosses . . . and that's just for openers!

The central character of the story is a beautiful, young virgin, the winner of the "Miss Persia Pageant." Well, actually she won a little more than a beauty pageant; it was a contest to find a replacement for King

Xerxes's wife. The king, also known as Ahasuerus, had recently banished his queen for insubordination. The king's attendants suggested the beauty pageant to find the king the most beautiful bride in the land, and the king bought the idea.

A fellow named Mordecai was Esther's older cousin and guardian. The cousins were of Jewish descent, living in the foreign land of Persia. Esther's name in Hebrew was "Hadassah," which loosely translates to "Myrtle" in English. Esther decided to stick with her Persian name, which means "a star."

And she was a star! The Bible calls attention to the fact that "the young lady was beautiful of form and face" (Esther 2:7). So Mordecai had a wild idea. Why not enter Esther in the king's competition?

When I entered the Miss Florida and Miss America pageants, my sponsoring committee helped me by putting me through several months of intensive preparation. It was fun, but it was tough, too. Still, I didn't go through anything compared to the prepping the king's attendants put Esther through!

For twelve months, they worked on her, night and day, just to get her ready for her debut before the king. An entire staff of maids monitored her daily diet and exercise program. Her beautification process consisted of a six-month treatment with myrrh and expensive, fragrant oil, followed by another six months of pampering with spices and other cosmetics (2:12). Whew! Talk about a beauty regimen. This girl had one!

When it came time for the contestants to parade before the king and his attendants, they were permitted to ask for anything they thought might enhance their chances—perfumes, designer clothes (actually, they were all "designer clothes" in the king's palace), or even

Many people spend their entire life indefinitely preparing to live.
PAUL TOURNIER
THE ADVENTURE OF LIVING

expensive jewelry (no word on whether they had to give back the clothes and jewelry after the contest). Nothing was too good for the king's potential queen.

Amazingly, Esther asked for nothing extra when she went in to see King Ahasuerus. She stood before the mightiest ruler on earth, adorned in the graces of a godly woman, what the apostle Peter years later referred to as "the imperishable quality of a gentle and quiet spirit, which is precious in the sight of God" (I Peter 3:4). But her natural beauty, charm, and grace blew the king away! Ahasuerus loved her and crowned her Queen of Persia.

I won't ruin the story for you by telling you the whole thing, but let's just say that Esther and her people had a problem. His name was Haman, sort of an intolerably arrogant, manipulative, "big man on campus type."

Haman hatched a plot to have all of the Jews who were living in Persia annihilated, and King Ahasuerus unwittingly gave the holocaust his approval. Little did Haman or the king know that Queen Esther was of Jewish ethnic background!

I'll let you read the rest of the story (it's just getting good!), but I'll give you a hint. By using a combination of her beauty, brains, and boldness, Esther turned the tables on the creep, Haman.

Not that she wasn't scared. She was! But her cousin Mordecai reminded her that God had given her everything she had: her looks; her position; her opportunity to make a difference in the lives of her family, her people, and all of history. His words were both a warning and an encouragement to her:

There is only one kind of beauty that can transcend time, and many women possess it. It is, of course, beauty of the spirit that lights the eyes and transforms even a plain woman into a beautiful one. Women with wit, charm, and warmth, who are interested in others and forget themselves, and who accept each stage of life gracefully, are the lasting beauties of this world—and the happiest.

DEIRDRE BUDGE

Seek first his kingdom and his righteousness, and all these things will be given to you as well.

MATTHEW 6:33 (NIV)

For if you remain silent at this time, relief and deliverance will arise for the Jews from another place and you and your father's house will perish. And who knows whether you have not attained royalty for such a time as this? (Esther 4:14)

Finally, Esther decided to take the ultimate risk. She placed her life on the line and said, "I will go . . . and if I perish, I perish" (4:16). Esther's courage saved her own life as well as the lives of her people. It also scuttled Haman's plot and spelled doom for that self-serving rascal. In addition, her cousin Mordecai was exalted to the position of prime minister. Myrtle did good!

I bring up this story at the end of this book because I think it shows us several key points to keep in mind every time we look in the mirror.

1. God knows where you are. He hasn't forgotten you. Sure, there may be days when you feel as though God is a zillion miles away, but He's not. He is right there with you, only a prayer away. Your time, like Esther's, will come.

2. You have a responsibility to take care of your body, not for proud, selfish reasons, but so you can present a worthy representation of, and to, the King of kings, the Lord Jesus. Esther had to work on her physical appearance all year before she went in before the king—and remember, she was already a beautiful young woman to begin with! That says to me that I should take my personal appearance seriously. No, you don't have to look like a beauty queen in order to live for or be accepted by Jesus. But living for Jesus is no excuse to be lazy about our looks, either. In fact, we should do our best to be as outwardly attractive as possible. God can bless,

honor, and use your physical beauty. Good grooming can bring glory to God.

3. You also have a responsibility to use your brains! Although Esther's beauty got her in the door, it was her bold, decisive thinking that won the day. She had studied the secular power system of which she had become a part. She knew how things worked in that volatile political climate. But she was also a student of human personality. She knew what made people tick and she used a little psychology, sociology, and philosophy to bring down the enemy.

   In her case, it was literally a "use your head or lose it" situation. While your immediate circumstances may not be so dire, the ultimate price is the same.

4. External beauty is insufficient without inner beauty. To me, this is the most impressive part of Esther's story. Pagan, secular people recognized that there was something different about Esther. The Scripture says that "Esther found favor in the eyes of all who saw her" (2:15), and those people were not in the habit of handing out compliments freely. I believe that what set Esther apart from all the other pretty shapes and faces was a radiance that only comes from a personal relationship with God.

Do you have that kind of relationship? If you don't, the best makeup will not bring about the inner beauty that is missing. Only Jesus can provide that. It is a natural, joyful result of trusting Him, of repenting of, and receiving forgiveness for, your sins, and of having Jesus at the center of your life. You can't conjure up inner beauty. You can't fake it. You can only receive it as part of God's free gift to you.

Let us, therefore, be ambitious of the wisdom of Solomon, rather than the glory of Solomon, in which he was outdone by the lilies. Knowledge and grace are the perfection of man, not beauty. . . .

NOTE ON MATTHEW 6:28, 29

MATTHEW HENRY

MATTHEW HENRY'S COMMENTARY ON THE WHOLE BIBLE

If you have never invited Jesus to come in and take control of your life, or if you are not totally sure, let me encourage you to do so right now. He's been my best friend for years. I guarantee you, He'll be the best friend you will ever have.

If you are serious about allowing Jesus to give you an inner make-over, you can pray a prayer something like this:

> *Heavenly Father,*
>
> *There's a bunch I don't understand just yet, and to tell You the truth, I'm a little nervous about this whole thing. But, I know that I believe in You. I want to belong to You, from now on. Please forgive my sins and make me over completely, from the inside out!*
>
> *Thank You, Lord, for forgiving me and for giving me a fresh beginning. I pray this in the name of Jesus, and for Your glory. Amen.*

If you sincerely prayed this prayer, Jesus Christ has come into your life. This is the most important step you will ever take. It's a brand-new life! Clean. Pure. Totally forgiven. Made over by the One who made you.

But it's not the end. It is just the beginning. There is so much more Jesus wants to do in and through and for you! Get yourself a Bible and check out Jesus' story in the Gospel of John. Read a bit from God's Word every day, and talk to Him in prayer. Also, please find a church where the people love Jesus, and where you can grow stronger in Him.

One more thing: Tell somebody else, or a bunch of somebodies, about your new relationship with Christ. You can start by telling me. I'd love to hear from you, so drop me a note in the mail (Kim Boyce, P.O. Box

I believe in the sun even when it is not shining. I believe in love even when I am not feeling it. I believe in God even when He is silent.

INSCRIPTION FROM A CELLAR IN COLOGNE, GERMANY, WHERE JEWS HAD BEEN HIDDEN DURING THE HOLOCAUST

121034, Nashville, TN 37212) and let me know how the Lord is making you over and how I can pray for you. I'm not interested in getting fan mail; I really want to hear from you, if you have trusted Jesus as a result of this book.

INNER BEAUTY—IT LASTS A LIFETIME

The other day I read an article about one of the former top models in the world who couldn't find work in her career. She was over the hill they said. Finished. Washed up. She was barely thirty years of age.

That article reminded me once more of a principle taught in the Bible: "Charm is deceitful and beauty is vain, but a woman who fears the Lord, she shall be praised" (Proverbs 31:30). Shortly after I had been crowned Miss Florida, I saw living proof of that.

While I was reigning as Miss Florida, I was invited to sing at a Christian college during a week of services honoring women in ministry. I arrived, feeling quite confident, "looking my best." I was wearing my favorite outfit, my makeup was just right, and my "beauty queen hairdo" was in top form.

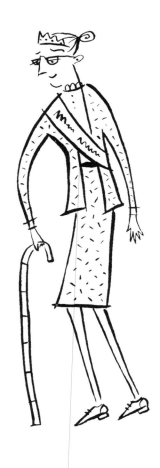

My time to sing finally came, and I took the stage and did my best to "bless" the crowd. After singing several songs, I sat down, thinking, "Hey, that was pretty good!"

But something happened in the next five minutes that I will never forget as long as I live.

The featured speaker was introduced, and she hobbled to the podium. She was eighty years old and walked very slowly in her orthopedic shoes. She was wearing a plain, navy-blue suit, a high-necked blouse, and her unadorned hair was pulled into a tight bun on top of her head.

When I first saw her, I thought she looked like a

You look at me
and see
my flaws;
I look at you
and see
flaws, too.
Those who love,
know love
deserves
a second glance;
each failure serves
another chance.
Love looks to see,
beyond the scars
and flaws,
the cause;
and scars become
an honorable badge
of battles fought
and won—
(or lost)
but fought!
The product,
not the cost,
is what love sought.
RUTH BELL GRAHAM

SITTING BY MY LAUGHING FIRE

sweet little grandmotherly type. Yet, as that lady began speaking, I realized who the real beauty queen was that night. She was the winner . . . and I didn't even place!

That dear woman told how she had been involved in mission work in Africa for more than forty years. For the first twenty years, she had labored with her loving husband. Then he went home to be with the Lord. After his death, she had faithfully carried on for another twenty years.

As the woman spoke to the audience, the Lord was speaking to me. The more she told of her story, the more shame I felt for having placed so much emphasis and value on my outward appearance that day. I promised the Lord, right then and there, while the former missionary was still speaking, that I would try to never again sacrifice inner beauty for outward adornment.

Someday, if the Lord tarries and allows me to continue serving Him, I will grow old, too. My hair will turn gray and may even start to fall out. I'll probably get wrinkles and walk a bit more slowly. And do you know what? So will you! It's inevitable.

There's nothing wrong with taking care of your outward appearance. In fact, as I've said all along, I believe there is a lot right about it. If I thought otherwise, I wouldn't have written an entire book about beauty. I sincerely hope that you will benefit from the beauty tips I have shared.

Yet it is important to me that you know that all of these hints and helps are given against the backdrop of the priceless beauty secret I learned from that little missionary lady. I never even got her name—she could have been an angel for all I know—but I will always be grateful to her for the lesson she taught me . . . and didn't even know it!

Nowadays, when people hear my name, they may recognize me as a recording artist. A few may remember me as one of many former Miss Floridas. But when the day comes for me to put on those orthopedic shoes, I want to be known as someone with inner beauty, someone who values the truly important things in life, someone who has known, loved, and served the Lord Jesus Christ!

How about you?

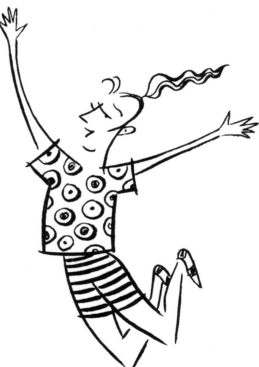

NOTES FROM TEXT

CHAPTER 2—FACE TO FACE

1. Victoria Principal, *The Beauty Principal* (New York, N.Y.: Simon & Schuster, 1984), 39.

CHAPTER 3—THREE SIMPLE STEPS TO SENSATIONAL SKIN

1. From *The New Medically Based No-Nonsense Beauty Book* by Deborah Chase. Copyright © 1989 by Deborah Chase. Reprinted by permission of Henry Holt and Company, Inc.
2. Eileen Ford, *Book of Model Beauty* (New York, N.Y.: Simon & Schuster, 1968), 116.

CHAPTER 4—MAXIMUM MASKS AND FANTASTIC FACIALS

1. Laura Lynn McCarthy, "Images: The Beauty Mask," *Vogue*; (Sept. 1990): 356.

CHAPTER 5—BREAKOUT BREAKTHROUGH

1. Adrien Arpel, *3-Week Makeover Shapeover Beauty Program* (New York, N.Y.: Rawson Associate Publishers, Inc., 1977), 32.

CHAPTER 6—SAY GOOD-BYE TO MR. SUNSHINE!

1. Chase, *The New Medically Based No-Nonsense Beauty Book*, 126.

CHAPTER 8—NO BODY IS PERFECT

1. Steve Silva "Facts on Fat," *Seventeen*; (May, 1990): 96.
2. Janis Graham, "The Great Diet Docs," *Harper's Bazaar*; (July, 1991): 74.
3. Ruth Lahmayer, M.S., R.D., "Seventeen's Guide to Healthy Weight Loss," *Seventeen*; (May, 1990): 79.
4. Scott Weigle, M.D., "Diet, Q & A," *Mademoiselle*; (June, 1990): 46.

CHAPTER 9—BUT I HATE TO EXERCISE!

1. Jennifer MacLeod, "Arnold Pumps You Up," *Seventeen*; (August, 1991): 158.